CARDIOLOGY RESEARCH AND CLINICAL DEVELOPMENTS

CORONARY ARTERY DISEASE

CHARACTERISTICS, MANAGEMENT AND LONG-TERM OUTCOMES

CARDIOLOGY RESEARCH AND CLINICAL DEVELOPMENTS

Additional books in this series can be found on Nova's website under the Series tab.

Additional e-books in this series can be found on Nova's website under the e-books tab.

CARDIOLOGY RESEARCH AND CLINICAL DEVELOPMENTS

CORONARY ARTERY DISEASE

CHARACTERISTICS, MANAGEMENT AND LONG-TERM OUTCOMES

COURTNEY BURKE
EDITOR

New York

Library of Congress Cataloging-in-Publication Data

ISBN: 978-1-63485-330-9
Library of Congress Control Number: 2016939458

Published by Nova Science Publishers, Inc. † New York

CONTENTS

PREFACE

Coronary artery disease (CAD) is a leading cause of mortality and morbidity worldwide. In approximately half of the patients with newly diagnosed CAD, the first presentation is either acute myocardial infarction or sudden cardiac death. This book provides current research on the characteristics, management and long-term outcomes of coronary artery disease. Chapter One begins with an overview of biological characteristics, clinical classification, and spasms of arterial grafts and antispastic management in coronary artery bypass grafting surgery. Chapter Two discusses coronary artery bypass grafting (CABG) and percutaneous coronary intervention (PCI) in the current era, and highlights relative strengths and weaknesses of each approach. It also discusses various risk-stratification scoring systems, and consider both procedures in the context of different demographic populations, including advanced age, gender, acute coronary syndromes, previous CABG, renal failure, diabetes mellitus and left main involvement. Chapter Three focuses on contribution facts and fables of gender disparities in cardiovascular diseases. Chapter Four examines the role of multi-detector computed tomography in the detection of subclinical coronary atherosclerosis in patients without known CAD.

Chapter 1 – CABG surgery has been the standard treatment for patients with coronary artery disease, particularly for three-vessel disease, although PCI has become the preferred method in one- or two-vessel disease. Arterial grafting using autologous arteries as the bypass grafts has been demonstrated to have superior long-term results. Arterial grafts can be classified Type I, II, and III for clinical consideration according to their biological characteristics. Use of the left internal mammary artery to graft the diseased LAD has become the standard method for almost all CABG surgery and bilateral IMA grafts may further enhance survival over the long-term. The radial artery is also commonly used as a bypass graft, and occasionally the right gastroepiploic artery, and inferior epigastric artery. However, in comparison to vein grafts, arterial grafts have a tendency to develop vasospasm that can lead to potentially life-threatening complications. Various antispastic pharmacologicals have been used during surgery but the rationale and efficacy are sometimes unclear and there is still controversy as to what is the most effective regimen. This is partially due to the pathophysiological complexity of the mechanism of vascular spasm and, consequently, the evolution of several pharmacological vasodilators. Better understanding of the mechanism of vascular spasm, development of new pharmacological vasodilators, and the adequate evaluation of non-pharmacological methods may lead to a more unanimous opinion as to the best method to prevent and treat arterial spasm in contemporary clinical practice.

Chapter 2 – Coronary artery disease is a leading cause of morbidity and mortality in developed countries around the globe. Coronary revascularization, either with coronary artery bypass grafting (CABG) or percutaneous coronary intervention (PCI) has been shown to be safe and effective in appropriately selected patients. Both revascularization strategies have undergone significant advancements, creating the need to (re) examine data from clinical studies and critically scrutinize existing guidelines in order to determine the optimal care for each individual patient. In this chapter, we will discuss the CABG and PCI in the current era, and highlight relative strengths and weaknesses of each approach. The authors will also discuss various risk-stratification scoring systems, and consider both procedures in the context of different demographic populations, including advanced age, gender, acute coronary syndromes, previous CABG, renal failure, diabetes mellitus and left main involvement. The continued development of objective patient-assessment tools to offer patient-tailored recommendation is critical. Moreover, novel therapeutic approaches and treatment regimens, such as a hybrid strategy, as well as techniques targeted at improving stent and graft patency will be evaluated. This synthesis of information will provide an essential framework for evidence-based approach of coronary revascularization in the current era and beyond.

Chapter 3 – Cardiovascular disease (CVD) affects men and women equally. Yet CVD is considered as a “Man’s Disease”. The patho-physiology of CVD differs significantly between the sexes. Thus American College of Cardiology (2011) laid specific guidelines focusing on women specific CVD prevention, diagnosis, management, treatment and outcomes. Compared to men, women are under-prevented, under-diagnosed, under-treated and under-studied with respect to CVD. Although women share similar risk factors like age, hypertension, diabetes, hyperlipidemia, obesity, family history of CVD with men; women specific variables like depression, pre-eclampsia, gestational diabetes, thyroid disease, psoriasis, gout and auto immune disorders contribute significantly. Besides, inflammatory markers suggesting risk of disease like high sensitivity C reactive protein are higher in women at baseline then men. Estrogen and progesterone are more influential in women; menstruation can affect hematologic and electrocardiographic indices; women have reduced sympathetic and enhanced parasympathetic activity. In response to stress, women experience an increased pulse rate, resulting in an increased cardiac output; men result in increased vascular resistance resulting in increased blood pressure. Difference in pain perception exists between sexes, resulting in variability in presenting symptoms. Women are more likely to attribute their symptoms to non cardiac causes complicating timely treatment. Recent acute coronary syndrome registries have shown that on admission women are less likely to receive heparin, ACE inhibitors, glycoprotein IIa/IIIb inhibitors; at discharge less likely to be prescribed aspirin and statin therapy. Women experience more drug related adverse events than men. Many specific areas of CVD like heart failure, atrial fibrillation, valvular and structural disease, peripheral vascular and cerebro-vascular disease should be examined for existing gender differences. The healthcare sector holds a very critical and contributing role in education of adult female subjects towards risks of CVD; women specific contributing factors; warning signs; strategies to avoid delay in treatment; promote adherence to lifestyle interventions; ensure proper dosage adjustments to reduce risk of bleeding and other adverse events; promote primary and secondary prevention guidelines; improve application of evidence based therapy to improve women care in CVD.

Chapter 4 – Coronary artery disease (CAD) is a leading cause of mortality and morbidity worldwide. In approximately half of the patients with newly diagnosed CAD, the first presentation is either acute myocardial infarction or sudden cardiac death. Moreover, approximately half of those developing CAD have been classified as having low or intermediate risk on the basis of a current risk algorithm. Recent studies have demonstrated that the major determinant of risk for atherosclerotic cardiovascular disease in asymptomatic adults is the presence of the underlying disease itself, namely subclinical atherosclerosis. Thus, it is essential to detect subclinical CAD before the manifestation of clinical CAD events.

Multi-detector computed tomography (MDCT) is a promising modality to evaluate CAD. MDCT has an excellent capacity to detect hemodynamically relevant stenosis and vulnerable plaque (also called high-risk plaque). Thus, the authors reviewed the studies that investigated the prevalence and characteristics of CAD in patients without known CAD by using MDCT.

These studies demonstrated that the prevalence of subclinical CAD in asymptomatic patients with low to intermediate risk was high, and that a substantial number of patients had significant stenosis. On the other hand, the prevalence of non-calcified plaque in asymptomatic patients with no or mild coronary calcium was relatively low, and significant coronary stenosis was rare in these patients.

Among diabetic patients, approximately two-thirds had subclinical CAD. The prevalence of significant stenosis and high-risk plaque, namely high-risk CAD, was significantly higher in these patients compared with that in those without diabetes. Moreover, some clinical characteristics could predict diabetic patients with high-risk CAD. In stroke patients, approximately two-thirds had subclinical CAD and one-fifth had high-risk CAD. The prevalence of high-risk CAD was two-fold higher in stroke patients compared with that in non-stroke patients. Patients with mild to moderate chronic kidney disease (CKD) had higher prevalence of significant stenosis and coronary plaque than did those without CKD. However the prevalence of high-risk plaque was not significantly different between the two groups. About three-quarters of patients with carotid artery disease had subclinical CAD, and higher intima-media thickness was associated with high-risk CAD.

Statin treatment is a mainstay of the treatment of patients with CAD. However, the study showed that CAD and carotid artery disease progressed significantly despite normal lipid values due to standard statin therapy in asymptomatic patients without known CAD. This suggests that more intense lipid lowering will be needed to prevent progression of CAD and carotid artery disease.

Taken together, these studies suggest that MDCT can detect subclinical CAD in patients with low to intermediate risk of but without known CAD, and that subclinical CAD is highly prevalent. The prevalence of high-risk CAD is particularly high in patients with diabetes, stroke, CKD, and carotid artery disease, but without known CAD. Intensive statin therapy is needed to prevent the progression of subclinical coronary atherosclerosis.

In: Coronary Artery Disease
Editor: Courtney Burke

ISBN: 978-1-63485-330-9

Chapter 1

BIOLOGICAL CHARACTERISTICS, CLINICAL CLASSIFICATION, AND SPASM OF ARTERIAL GRAFTS AND ANTISPASTIC MANAGEMENT IN CORONARY ARTERY BYPASS GRAFTING SURGERY

Guo-Wei He**, MD, PhD, DSc

TEDA International Cardiovascular Hospital,
Chinese Academy of Medical Sciences and Peking Union Medical College, Tianjin and The Affiliated Hospital of Hangzhou Normal University and Zhejiang University, Hangzhou, China,
Department of Surgery, Oregon Health and Science University, Portland, Oregon, US

ABSTRACT

CABG surgery has been the standard treatment for patients with coronary artery disease, particularly for three-vessel disease, although PCI has become the preferred method in one- or two-vessel disease. Arterial grafting using autologous arteries as the bypass grafts has been demonstrated to have superior long-term results. Arterial grafts can be

* Correspondence author. Address: No.61, the 3rd Ave., TEDA, Tianjin, 300457 or No. 126, Wenzhou Road, Hangzhou, Zhejiang, 310015, China. Tel: 86-22-6520 9089; Fax: 86-22-6520 8732; E-mail: gwhezj@163.com.

classified Type I, II, and III for clinical consideration according to their biological characteristics. Use of the left internal mammary artery to graft the diseased LAD has become the standard method for almost all CABG surgery and bilateral IMA grafts may further enhance survival over the long-term. The radial artery is also commonly used as a bypass graft, and occasionally the right gastroepiploic artery, and inferior epigastric artery. However, in comparison to vein grafts, arterial grafts have a tendency to develop vasospasm that can lead to potentially life-threatening complications. Various antispastic pharmacologicals have been used during surgery but the rationale and efficacy are sometimes unclear and there is still controversy as to what is the most effective regimen. This is partially due to the pathophysiological complexity of the mechanism of vascular spasm and, consequently, the evolution of several pharmacological vasodilators. Better understanding of the mechanism of vascular spasm, development of new pharmacological vasodilators, and the adequate evaluation of non-pharmacological methods may lead to a more unanimous opinion as to the best method to prevent and treat arterial spasm in contemporary clinical practice.

I. INTRODUCTION

CABG surgery has been the standard treatment for patients with coronary artery disease (CAD), particularly for three-vessel disease, although over the past decade, percutaneous coronary intervention (PCI) has gradually become the preferred method of revascularization in patients with one-vessel or two-vessel disease [1, 2]. Arterial grafting, i.e., using autologous arteries rather than veins as the grafts, has been demonstrated to have superior long-term results compared to vein grafts [3]. In particular, use of the left internal mammary artery (IMA) to graft the diseased LAD has become the standard method for almost all CABG surgery [4, 5]. In addition, other arteries such as the radial artery (RA) [6, 7], and less commonly the right gastroepiploic artery (GEA) [8-10], and the inferior epigastric artery (IEA) [11-12] are used as bypass grafts. However, arterial grafts are relatively small arteries with a varying muscular component in the vessel wall and have a tendency to develop vasospasm during surgery, as discussed below in details.

Antispastic therapy therefore has been and remains an important issue through the history of development of CABG particularly in arterial grafting. Studies of the pathophysiology of spasm and the development of antispastic pharmacological management have paralled the employment of arterial grafts in CABG [13-61]. This has included a large number of pharmacological and some non-pharmacological methods to prevent or treat vasospasm. Due to the complexity of the antispastic drugs and other methods involved, no single technique for antispastic management has been uniformly accepted or adopted. In this Review, we discuss the evidence base for the existence and incidence of vasospasm in CABG surgery using arterial grafts, the clinically available potential antispastic methods, and their possible advantages and disadvantages with a view to help elucidate mechanisms of vasospasm of arterial grafts and the decision making in choice of the potential antispastic methods.

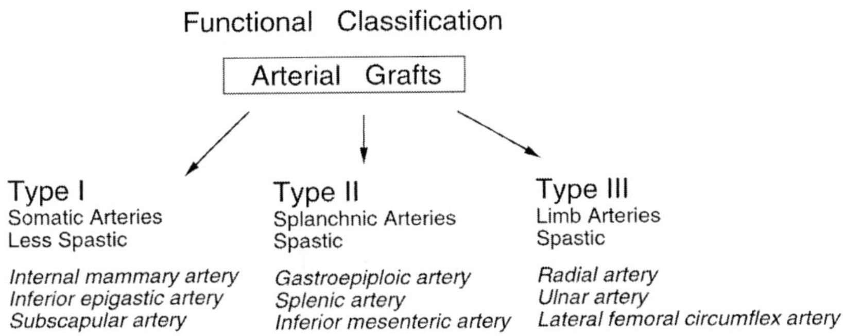

Figure 1. The functional classification for arterial grafts, often referred as "HE classification" (From He GW: Arterial grafts for coronary artery bypass grafting: biological characteristics, functional classification, and clinical choice. *Ann Thorac Surg*. 1999;67:277-84. With permission).

I.1. Biological Characteristics and Clinical Classification of Arterial Grafts

The biological characteristics of arterial grafts are the basis of the behavior when they are grafted on the coronary artery system. A clinical classification is useful for a practicing surgeon. Based on our own experimental studies on the vasoreactivity combined with anatomical, physiological, and embryological considerations of the arterial grafts, I have proposed a functional classification for the grafts, suggesting that there are three types of arterial grafts: Type I- somatic arteries; Type II- splanchnic arteries; and Type III- limb arteries [29, 62]. The Type I arteries have better endothelial function and release more nitric oxide and other vasorelaxing factors [63, 64]; the Type II arteries, such as the gastro-epiploic artery, and the Type III arteries, such as the radial artery, have higher pharmacological reactivity to vasoconstrictors.

The Type III arteries were later demonstrated to have higher contractility [65] and less eNOS expression [66]. This classification explains why the IMA has the best long-term patency. Because Type II and III arteries are prone to spasms due to higher contractility, they require more active pharmacological interventions.

II. Pathophysiology of Spasm

II.1. Existence and Incidence of Spasm of Arterial Grafts

Prevalence of Spasm of IMA

Spasm of IMA was first reported in 1987 [48]. Spasm could be a localized phenomenon or a diffuse process, referred to as a "string sign"[49], could cause hypoperfusion, typically occurring 30 to 40 minutes after discontinuation of cardiopulmonary bypass but also seen subsequently in the intensive care unit [50] when it may also be confused with coronary artery spasm. IMA spasm may also occur years after bypass grafting [51].

Based on these clinical observations, a large body of studies has been reported on the physiological and pharmacological characteristics of the IMA to understand the nature of spasm. In an early study, I demonstrated that the contractility of the distal section of the IMA is inversely correlated to its diameter; that is, the smaller the diameter, the greater the tendency for spasm to develop. This suggests that trimming off the distal end of the IMA as much as possible may be the best way to prevent graft spasm [52]. Nevertheless, since 1980s, a large body of literature has demonstrated the existence of spasm in IMA even in current practice [53-60].

The exact incidence of spasm of arterial grafts is unknown. This is particularly due to the fact that when it is mild, it may be asymptomatic; or, if responsible to vasodilator treatment, it is usually not reported. However, when spasm is severe and has little response to the usual pharmacological management, it can be lethal [53-57, 59]. A recent report indicated that among 5,762 patients who underwent isolated CABG, 7 patients (0.12%) experienced refractory spasm of coronary arteries and grafted conduits including the left IMA and 18 patients experienced perioperative vasospasm of a single coronary artery or of a grafted conduit [59]. This suggests that the confirmed severe perioperative vasospasm in coronary artery of grafts is about 0.43% in all CABG surgery. It is possible that the incidence of vasospasm could be underestimated because there could be some patients who have vasospasm responsible to early use of vasodilator agents and not counted as vasospasm.

The Incidence of Spasm in Other Arterial Grafts

The RA and GEA have been demonstrated as prone to spasm. Dramatically, the revival of the use of RA was due to the use of successful antispastic management [6]. Since the more widespread use of the RA, spasm has been reported more frequently by cardiac surgeons [67], physicians [68] and cardiologists during catheterization [69]. Gabe and colleagues reported an unusual case of CABG, complicated by vasospasm of a grafted RA leading to postoperative ventricular fibrillation. RA graft spasm was demonstrated by angiography and was successfully resolved by intravenous nitroglycerin administration [70]. In addition, focal RA graft stenosis may be difficult to differentiate from spasm and can be treated by percutaneous intervention [71].

GEA spasm is also a well-recognized complication. Spasm can occur during or soon after harvesting of these vasoreactive grafts [72-74] or a few months or years postoperatively, as demonstrated by angiography [75].

There are fewer reports on IEA spasm. This is probably due to the fact that first, anatomically and functionally, IEA belongs to the Type I artery that may be less spastic [29, 62, 76] and second, use of IEA is not as frequent as IMA, RA, or GEA. However, occasionally, IEA graft is reported to have spasm even at 5-year angiographic follow-up [61].

II.2. Mechanisms of Spasm of Arterial Grafts

Despite of the efforts to try to understand the mechanism(s) of vascular spasm, it is still not fully understood owing to the complex nature at molecular levels. However, it is understood that spasm is an extreme form of vasoconstriction. In general, vasoconstriction may be evoked by a number of stimulants. Mechanical stimulation, nerve stimulation, as well as vasoconstrictor substances are common stimulants of vasoconstriction [17, 77]. These vasoconstrictor substances are therefore referred to as spasmogens. The possible spasmogens in arterial grafts have been well studied. These include: endothelium-derived contracting factors such as endothelin-1 [77, 78], prostaglandins such as TX_{A2} or mimetics and $PGF_{2\alpha}$, α-adrenoceptor agonists such as norepinephrine, methoxamine and phenylephrine, platelet-derived substances such as 5-HT, and cellular membrane depolarizing agent potassium [77], mast cells and histamine [79]. It should be noted that studies have been performed in the human vessels since there are marked differences between human and animal vessels in response to these spasmogens [15, 17]. In addition, there are differences in responses between the IMA and coronary artery to vasoconstrictors [29]. In general, arterial grafts have higher responsiveness to norepinephrine because the coronary artery is α- and β-adrenoceptor-balanced vessel. However, IMA [19, 21, 80] and RA [37] are α-adrenoceptor predominant vessels. On the other hand, however, it has also been demonstrated that IMA graft is unresponsive to ergonovine at least in the amount required to produce coronary artery spasm in patients with variant angina [81]. In comparison to the IMA and IEA, the GEA has been demonstrated to have highest responsiveness to endothelin, TXA_2 mimetic, and potassium [29]. Subsequently, RA was demonstrated to have higher receptor-mediated contractility to endothelin and angiotensin II [65], vasopressin [82], 5-HT [83], and TXA_2 [84].

Other causes for vasospasm in arterial grafts may be related to certain pathways of vascular contractility or endothelial dysfunction. For example, autologous neutrophils release a stable non-protein small molecule that disturbs internal mammary artery endothelial function [85]. In addition, it was demonstrated that RhoA/Rho kinase pathway may be one mechanism by which RA is more susceptible to spasm than IMA [86] and that isoprostane responses in radial arteries are found to be mediated by prostanoid receptors selective for TXA_2 with activation of Rho-kinase and release of Ca^{2+} [87].

Recently, it has been recognized that fat cells or adipocytes produce large numbers of metabolically active substances with both endocrine and paracrine actions. Perivascular adipose tissue may play a role in the mechanism of vascular spasm [88].

Apart from vasoconstrictor spasmogens, other stimulants such as hypothermia [89] have also been demonstrated to be related to spasm of the grafts. Metabolic diseases such as diabetes mellitus have been demonstrated to increase the risk of radial artery spasm [67].

It must be indicated that the intact endothelium plays an extremely important role to prevent vascular spasm. The endothelium releases a number of endothelium-derived relaxing factors such as nitric oxide (NO), endothelium-derived hyperpolarizing factor, and PGI_2 [33, 34, 36] that keeps the adequate vascular tone in the arterial grafts. This is why it is ultimately important to prevent endothelial damage when using arterial grafts.

III. PHARMACOLOGICAL MANAGEMENT FOR SPASM (PHARMACOLOGICAL ANTISPASTIC METHODS)

Pharmacological studies have paralleled the development of the arterial grafts in CABG [17-28] owing to the fact that arterial grafts are relatively small arteries and there is a tendency to develop spasm in these arteries during surgery, as described above. Pharmacological studies on CABG grafts were initially focused on the IMA. Along with the increased use of other arterial grafts, studies have been also extended to these arteries. Pharmacological management in CABG is a complex topic. It should actually include two aspects. This may involve firstly, systematic use of pharmacological agents in order to maintain cardiac output and graft function during the pre-, intra-, and post-operative period, and secondly, specific pharmacological management for arterial conduits by using both systematic and topical methods.

Adequate understanding of the mechanism of vasoconstriction and the effect of vasodilators is essential to design any protocols to use vasodilators. Such understanding should be based on 1). the nature of vasoconstriction and the mechanism of the vasodilators [77]; 2). the status of the contraction that refers to prevent or to reverse existing contraction/spasm [17]; 3). duration of the use of a vasodilator agent, which refers to single or long-term use; the latter may develop tolerance such as to nitrates [90]. The role of mitochondrial aldehyde dehydrogenase was discovered [90], which specifically generates 1,2-glyceryl dinitrate from nitroglycerin, in the bioactivation of nitroglycerin to elicit vasorelaxation and in the development of tolerance to nitroglycerin; 4). the concentration of vasodilator that should be correlated to the plasma concentrations if used systematically but could be much higher if used topically [17]; and 5) the rapidity of onset of effect that may maximally relief spasm [14, 24].

III.1. The Vasodilator Agents Used for Arterial Grafts

Papaverine. Papaverine is a traditional topical vasodilator and is probably a pharmacological vasodilator used earlier than most others. The satisfactory results were reported in early studies [91]. Papaverine is an opioid-derivative and a non-specific vasodilator substance, which relaxes blood vessels through multiple mechanisms. It is a phosphodiesterase inhibitor and therefore may raise cGMP level in smooth muscle cells [92]. Papaverine-induced relaxation is also due to other actions such as decreased calcium influx [93], or inhibition of release of intracellularly stored calcium [94]. It usually relaxes vessels (such as human IMA) at high concentrations regardless of the nature of the contraction. It has been suggested that papaverine has a satisfactory vasorelaxant effect in IMA [91, 95-100] and other arterial grafts [101]. However, papaverine is not recommended for systemic use. The major concern of the topical use of papaverine is its acidic nature (pH 4.4 at -2.6 log M and pH 4.8 at -4.5 log M [23], which may damage the endothelial function. These concentrations are related to the solutions used for surgery as demonstrated in the human RA [36]. A common clinical protocol to topically use papaverine is to mix papaverine with blood. This may reduce its acidity due to the buffering effect of blood. On the other hand, papaverine hydrochloride is relatively unstable in non-acidic solutions and a white precipitate sometimes formed when papaverine is added to plasmalyte solution (pH approximately 7.4) [13] and the effect of this phenomenon in papaverine-blood mixture is unknown. In addition, the onset of vasodilation effect of papaverine is slower than other vasodilators such as NTG and verapamil although once reaches the plateau, the effect of papaverine is sustained [23, 34]. Papaverine was also shown to be inferior to nitroglycerin in GEA [102].

Nitrovasodilators. Organic nitrates (nitrovasodilators) such as nitroglycerin (NTG, i.e., glyceryl trinitrate [GTN]), sodium nitroprusside (SNP), or isosorbide dinitrate are widely used in CABG patients. The mechanism of vasorelaxation of these vasodilators is that they release NO, a powerful stimulant for guanylate cyclase which raises cGMP in the smooth muscle cell [103]. This subsequently reduces intracellular calcium concentrations and leads to relaxation of the smooth muscle cell.

Nitrovasodilators (NTG or SNP) have been demonstrated to be potent vasodilators in the human IMA [17, 20, 23, 25, 33, 41, 42, 44, 45, 47, 104-109], RA [36, 38, 41, 42, 44, 45, 106-108, 110], GEA [40, 105], and IEA [30, 106]. It was demonstrated that NTG is effective for either topical [19, 42, 102, 109, 110] or systemic [42, 44, 107] use. Nitrates are slightly more effective in blocking receptor-operated channels than blocking depolarizing agent-mediated contraction [17]. Early studies focusing on NTG and nitroprusside showed different effects of these drugs in vitro and in vivo [104]. Another group of NO donors thionitrites such as S-nitrosothiol RIG200 has been demonstrated to have prolonged, NO-mediated relaxation [111].

Importantly, nitrates are effective in treating established vascular spasm, regardless of the nature of the contraction; i.e., they are effective in reversing either receptor-mediated (TXA_2 receptors, adrenoceptors, or ET receptors) contraction or depolarizing agent (K^+)-mediated contraction [17]. However, they are less potent in prevention of vasospasm [17, 19, 20, 38]. This is probably related to the tolerance of a vessel to these nitrovasodilators [19, 25, 90, 103], as demonstrated later that mitochondrial aldehyde dehydrogenase plays a role in the mechanism of the development of tolerance to nitroglycerin [90]. Compared each other, NTG is more potent than SNP in the vasorelaxing effect but SNP is more effective in preventing ANGII and α-adrenoceptor-mediated contraction in the IMA [35].

Calcium antagonists. Classical calcium antagonists were three chemically divergent groups - dihydropyridine (nifedipine, exc.), phenylalkylamines (verapamil, exc.), and benzothiazepines (diltiazem, exc.). The new generations of these drugs, particularly the new dihydropyridines such as nisoldipine [112], nicardipine [113-116], amlodipine [117], cilnidipine [118], and azalnidipine [119], have been developed in the past decades and their effect on arterial grafts have been investigated. In general, they all express vasodilatory effect in arterial grafts. In addition to the calcium channel blockage, some of these new generations of calcium antagonists such as amlodipine [117], cilnidipine [118], and azalnidipine [119] may also stimulate the vascular endothelium to release NO that may further enhance the vasorelaxant effect in arterial grafts. It is possible that these new vasodilators may be proved to be usefeul in the prevention of spasm in arterial grafts.

In fact, calcium antagonists have been used as antispastic drugs in arterial grafting either alone [6, 120] or in combination to NTG [23, 34, 36, 39, 121]. Among the first generation of the three calcium antagonists, it was reported that diltiazem is the least potent one and nifedipine is 15-fold more potent than diltiazem in IMA [17]. However, diltiazem contributed to the successful revival of the RA after this graft was abandoned for almost 20-years due to serious spasm problems [6]. In contrast, diltiazem was reported to have little effect on human RA contractions [38, 43]. Further, verapamil is more potent than diltiazem in the human vessels [17] and this drug was available in injection form, therefore it was reconmmended to be included in the antispastic protocols [23, 34, 36]. As discussed before, in arterial grafts the effects of vasodilators depend on the nature of the vasoconstriction and this is particularly important for calcium antagonists. When IMA contracts with depolarizing agent potassium (K^+), nifedipine or other calcium antagonists are very effective in both preventing and reversing IMA contraction through inhibition of L-type calcium channel [17]. This is due to the fact that calcium antagonists relax blood vessels through a specific mechanism. Calcium antagonists reduce Ca^{2+} influx by blocking voltage-operated calcium channels, which is the major mechanism for the depolarizing agent K^+ to contract vessels. Therefore, calcium antagonists are particularly effective in preventing or treating K^+-induced contraction and this has been demonstrated in either IMA [17, 39] or RA [38, 43]. However, calcium antagonists such as nifedipine are less effective in contraction mediated by receptors such as TXA_2 receptors [17], α-adrenoceptors [27 122], ET [25, 123], or vasopressin (VP1 receptors) - mediated contraction [124].

Phosphodiesterase (PDE) inhibitors. As modulators of vascular smooth muscle tone, intracellular cAMP and cGMP are controlled through synthesis by cyclases and through hydrolysis by PDEs that are classified to at least five types. PDE III inhibitors such as amrinone or milrinone are known to inhibit cGMP-inhibitable low Km cAMP PDE [125]. The cardiac and vascular smooth muscle actions are favorable in postoperative management of patients who undergo open heart surgery, particularly in patients who present ventricular dysfunction and receive arterial grafts for CABG. The effect of PDEIII inhibitor milrinone on the IMA [33, 126, 127] or RA [82, 128, 129], and PDEIIIA inhibitor olprinone on the GEA and RA [130] has been studied and shown effective. It is noticed that the effect of milrinone on the IMA is superior to that on RA [82]. Further, in the systemic use, after cardiopulmonary bypass, milrinone dilates the IMA [131] and perioperative continuous infusion of milrinone, compared with nifedipine, results in a significantly lower incidence of myocardial ischaemia and myocardial cell damage after elective CABG [132]. In opposite, another PDEIII inhibitor enoximone is a potent in vitro vasodilator but exerts weak relaxant effects in IMA and GEA at concentrations in the therapeutic range [133].

α-adrenoceptor antagonists. It has been demonstrated that both IMA [21, 134] and RA [37, 134] are α_1-adrenoceptor-predominant artery. However, IMA has little α_2-adrenoceptor [21] whereas the RA has significant α_2-adrenoceptor [37] function, although the RA is also α_1-adrenoceptor predominant. This is the rationale to use α-adrenoceptor antagonists such as phenoxybenzamine as antispastic drug in CABG as an effective agent to prevent catecholamine-mediated spasm of RA [135, 136].

Phenoxybenzamine is reported more effective and less harmful than papaverine in the prevention of radial artery vasospasm [137, 138]. On the other hand, however, theoretically, α-adrenoceptor antagonists are only effective in reversing the contraction evoked by α-adrenoceptor but not to other vasoconstrictors as may be predicted from the pharmacological mechanism of α-adrenoceptor antagonists, i.e., α-adrenoceptor antagonists may only be effective in one specific mechanism of spasm and could be

the vascular smooth muscle cells into a relaxed state and reduce membrane excitability and the reactivity of the cell [158]. It has been suggested that vascular smooth muscle is particularly sensitive to KCOs [157]. Considering these characteristics, KCOs are of great value as therapeutical agents. Aprikalim [159, 160], levcromakalim [161, 162], KRN4884 [163], and rilmakalim [162] have been studied in the human IMA and found to be potent vasodilators in a number of receptor-mediated contraction and therefore, these KCOs may become a clinically useful antispastic drug in arterial grafts.

Antiplatelet drugs. Activated platelets induce pronounced contraction of the gastroepiploic artery that may contribute to postoperative spasm. Therefore vasodilators that prevent the effects of TXA_2 and serotonin may be beneficial to gastroepiploic artery graft function [164].

Vasodilators through other mechanisms potentially useful for antispastic protocols. A few of other substances have been investigated in the human arterial grafts and suggested be potential antispastic agents. Nutritional supplement L-carnitine Carnitine, a quaternary ammonium compound biosynthesized from the amino acids lysine and methionine, is widely available as a nutritional supplement. L-carnitine is a potential vasodilatory drug for internal mammary artery and saphenous vein grafts [165]. Botulinum toxin inhibits muscle contraction for about three months and is shown to prevented arterial graft spasm in vitro and had a longer lasting effect than papaverine, with no toxic effect on the artery of rats [166] but there were no human artery studies. Finally, NO-independent soluble guanylate cyclase (sGC) activator YC-1, and DEA/NO (diethylamine/nitric oxide), a NO-nucleophile adduct may be effective as vasodilator for the short-term treatment of perioperative spasm of coronary bypass grafts [167]. Most likely, those vasodilator substances would unlikely be primarily chosen as clinical antispastic agents.

Combination of vasodilators. It must be emphasized that all vasodilators have their own limitations in some aspect because each of them has a specific mechanism or mechanisms to relax vessels. These mechanisms have been discussed above. Combination of these vasodilators may overcome these disadvantages and therefore produce a better effect. Some of the combinations have been studied in the IMA and RA. For example, as an intraluminal or topical solution for the preparation of the grafts, calcium antagonists and NTG may have synergistic effect in IMA [23, 39, 112, 168] and in RA [34, 36 22, 23; 121, 169]. Yoshizaki and associates have demonstrated that combination of verapamil and nitroglycerin improves the patency rate of radial artery grafts [169]. Even in the critical situation with lethal spasm problems, the combination of NTG and verapamil has been reported to successfully release the spasm in arterial grafts through intraluminal injection that was a life salvage procedure [54]. The method is used successfully by others to relieve the coronary spasm as well [170] and is now used in catheterization laboratory for preventing RA spasm with success [171].

Other combination of vasodilators may also be clinically useful. The more than additive effect of milrinone and NTG has also been demonstrated [33] although such in vivo effect is to be demonstrated [46]. In addition, combined use of enoximone (a PDEIII inhibitor) and dobutamine (a beta-receptor agonist) at concentrations in the therapeutic range exerts a greater than additive vasorelaxant effect in IMA and GEA [133]. However, the role of such combination of vasodilator drugs in preparation of arterial grafts is to be established.

Taken together, from literature, the effect of a particular vasodilator in prevention or treatment of spasm in arterial grafts is often contradictory. We may conclude that there is no "perfect" vasodilator for dilating the IMA or other arterial grafts. This is due to the fact that spasm of arterial grafts may involve many mechanisms and each particular vasodilator may only relax the vessel through one mechanism or sometimes more than one mechanisms but no vasodilator may relax the vessel through all mechanisms. Under some circumstances, combination of vasodilators may be preferable.

Table 1. Summary of the antispastic protocols and existing techniques used in arterial grafting in CABG (from reference 202 with permission)

Authors	Topical	IMA	GEA	RA	Systemic	Postoperative oral
Mills 1989 [91]	papaverine	+				
Acar 1992 [6]	papaverine + blood			+	Diltiazem	Diltiazem
Suma 1991 [101]	papaverine		+			
Dietl 1995 [25]	papaverine			+	Diltiazem	Diltiazem "if spasm is noted"
Dregelid1995 [95]	papaverine	+				
Reyes 1995 [27]	papaverine 60 mg + 60 ml blood			+	Diltiazem	
Sasson 1995 [96]	papaverine	+				
Bilgen 1996 [97]	papaverine	+				
Yavuz 2001 [98]	papaverine	+				
Girard 2004 [99]	papaverine	+				
Tatoulis 2004	Papaverine			+	Nitroglycerin	amlodipine

Authors	Topical	IMA	GEA	RA	Systemic	Postoperative oral
[22]						
Bahcivan 2007 [100]	papaverine	+				
Kiessling 2013 [32]	Papaverine					
He GW 1994 [23]	VG	+				
He GW 1996 [34, 36]	VG			+#	Nicardipine*	one calcium antagonist**
Esmore 2000 [28]	VG			+	Nitroglycerin	
Yoshizaki 2008 [169]	VG			+#		
Mussa 2003 [135]	Phenoxy-benzamine			+		
Corvera 2003 [136]	Phenoxy-benzamine			+		
Gurevitch 1997 [106]	isosorbide dinitrate #	+	+	+		
Shapira 2000 [107]				+#	Nitroglycerin	
Chavanon 1999 [40]	Nitroglycerin		+			
García-Rinaldi 1999 [128]	milrinone			+		
Halpenny 2001 [143]		+			fenoldopam (D1 agonist)	
Zabeeda 2001 [44]		+#		+#	Nitroglycerin	
Möllhoff 2002 [132]				+#	milrinone	
Inokuchi 2004 [148]		+			Fasudil (through catheter)	
Tabel 2004 [120]		+			Diltiazem	
Nisanoglu 2006 [110]	Nitroglycerin			+		
Yamaguchi 2006 [130]	PDEIII inhibitor (olprinone)			+		
He 2008 [114]; Zheng 2012 [115]	NG	+			Nicardipine*	one calcium antagonist**
Ustunsoy 2009 [146]				+#	iloprost (5 days preop)	
Watanabe 2013 [149]	fasudil			+#		

III.2. Existing Pharmacological Methods (Antispastic Protocols) to Overcome Spasm

There are various antispastic protocols available in different units around the world.

Pharmacological methods are the most common antispastic protocols used in clinical practice world-widely.

Table 1 gives summary of the pharmacological antispastic protocols used in the practice of arterial grafting. Some of the protocols were designed based on the pharmacological studies on arterial grafts, as detailed in Table 1. However, other protocols are rather empirical.

IV. Non-Pharmacological Therapy to Overcome Spasm

IV.1. Denervation or Skeletonization or En-Bloc Harvesting?

It has been suggested that skeletonized arterial grafting may reduce the risk of graft spasm and may improve graft patency [172] and the removal of the periarterial sympathetic nerve from the human gastroepiploic artery reduced vascular contraction, elicited by peripheral nerve stimulation, without disturbing endothelial and smooth muscle contractile functions. This reduction may contribute to the prevention of vasospasms [10].

Similarly, it was reported that the results of using skeletonized radial artery grafts are excellent [130, 173-175] and this is often done with the ultrasonic scalpel [173, 174]. Kucukarslan and colleagues [176] used long fasciotomy of the posterior aspect of the RA for the purpose of sympathectomy to prepare the RA graft and believed this technique provides a satisfactory increase in the blood flow index and reduces the manipulation time as well as the risk of injury to the graft.

On the other hand, a study from Germany compared the skeletonization technique with pedicle preparation using either an ultrasonic scalpel or scissors and analyzed endothelial morphology by scanning electron microscopy and the conclusion is that skeletonization with an ultrasonic scalpel did not result in additional length and was more frequently associated with severe endothelial damage. Pedicle preparation using scissors or an ultrasonic scalpel is much simpler and faster, and does not jeopardize endothelial integrity [177].

Therefore, whether the skeletonization technique gives better results is still in debate.

In support of the above study, en-bloc free gastroepiploic artery graft, which has the gastroepiploic vein anastomosed to the right atrial appendage to prevent graft spasm [178] is proposed. They believed that the free gastroepiploic artery grafting with venous drainage technique can prevent graft spasm, leading to improved patency rate.

A retrospective review [179] in 57 patients who received en-bloc grafts and 29 who had skeletonized grafts reveals that 80-month patency rates of 100% for en-bloc grafts and 60% for skeletonized grafts. The observation, however, requires further clinical trials to be confirmed.

IV.2. Carbon Dioxide Insufflation

Carbon dioxide insufflation of the internal thoracic artery was suggested to be an efficient technique to increase the flow and prevent vasospasm [180]. The reactivity of the human internal mammary artery grafts harvested by either classical or carbon dioxide insufflation technique was compared; carbon dioxide insufflation technique does seem not only to protect the integrity of the endothelium and the whole vessel, but also prevent the possible vasospasm of the internal mammary artery segments [181].

IV.3. Normothermia or Heat Therapy or No Need for Vasodilators

Normothermia. It is possible that hypothermia plays an important role in radial artery vasospasm. It was even proposed that after harvesting the graft, regaining physiological normothermic state is enough for vasodilatation [182]. It has been suggested by the same group that preserving internal thoracic artery pedicles in normothermic conditions can be the preferred treatment for spasms [183] and that store of the radial artery graft in normothermic bath may relieve spasm of radial artery and the effect is similar to the use of verapamil-nitroglycerin solution [184]. On opposite, it was also proposed to treat radial artery grafts thermally in situ (45°C to 65°C; up to 120 s), so-called thermal ablation with effective anti-spastic effect [185].

However, the concept in those sporadic reports has not been widely accepted.

As mentioned above, the causes and mechanisms of vasospasm involve multiple factors, unlikely the temperature is the only factor affecting the vascular contraction/relaxation balance and therefore it is unlikely true that to use normothermia as the anti-spastic method would be effective under all situations.

IV.4. Injection of Room Air Beneath the Endothoracic Fascia Before IMA Dissection

Occasionally, injection of room air beneath the endothoracic fascia before IMA dissection is used to prevent spasm and shorten harvest time [186] but the practice is not widely accepted.

IV.5. Harmonic Scalpel

Since causes of vasospasm of the grafts may involve thermal injury caused by electrocautery and traumatic harvesting technique, the harmonic scalpel was proposed to decrease the harvesting time, frequency of spasm, and excessive use of hemostatic clips [187].

This technique was rapidly spread out and was demonstrated to be effective in harvesting of the RA associated with decreased RA spasm, good hemostasis, no additional harvest time, and has become standard technique in a number of units [188-193]. In addition, it was demonstrated that the optical coherence tomographic findings suggest that the harmonic scalpel induces less spasm and intimal injury compared with electrocautery [194].

IV.6. Intraoperative Detection of Intimal Lipid in the Radial Artery Predicts Degree of Postoperative Spasm

In two reports from one group [195, 196], optical coherence tomography imaging was used as a quality assurance tool for evaluating endoscopic harvest of the radial artery and the authors imaged RA conduits before and after CABG in order to characterize intimal abnormalities that might be related to the risk of spasm. They reported that the degree of attenuation of the optical coherence tomography (OCT) signal produced by the RA was strongly correlated with percentage diameter change and was significantly more pronounced in grafts with spasm versus no spasm. Histology confirmed lipid deposits in areas of RA with strong attenuation. RA conduits were often found by OCT imaging to have a substantial amount of lipid, which in turn strongly relates to the risk of postoperative spasm. Screening conduits based on characteristics of intimal quality may improve results following RA grafting [195] and catheter-based OCT provide an important quality assurance tool for RA harvest [196].

IV.7. Careful Dissection and Preparation of the IMA Pedicle to Prevent Injury and Spasm

Tector and colleagues [197] emphasize that initial flow in the IMA immediately after grafting is critical to the success of the operation. Careful dissection and preparation of the IMA pedicle to prevent injury and spasm, constructing parallel and perpendicular anastomoses so the most proximal portion of the IMA is used for anastomosis and the use of the free right IMA to increase length of graft available are measures employed to increase critical flow.

IV.8. Intractable LIMA Spasm in the Postoperative Period Treated by Placement of 'Bridging' Stent - A “Hybrid Procedure”

Pratt and colleagues [57] reported that a woman with critical left main stenosis suffered intractable left internal mammary artery (LIMA) spasm post-coronary artery bypass grafting. This was managed with a left main stent and the patient stabilized. A 3-month follow-up angiogram showed a patent graft and a blocked stent. This “hybrid”method may be the choice of the patients under such circumstances.

IV.9. Pre-Emptive Stellate Ganglion Block

Pre-emptive stellate ganglion block (SGB) was suggested to be an effective method for increasing radial artery blood flow and preventing radial artery spasm [198].

IV.10. Extrafascially Harvested Radial Artery

It was suggested that when the radial artery is harvested extrafascially, with diltiazem infusion, the RA may be used with improve the early and long-term results [199].

IV.11. Injection of Vasodilators into Arterial Grafts Through Cardiac Catheter to Relieve Spasm

When the grafts or the coronary artery develop spasm perioperatively, injection of vasodilators such as verapamil plus nitroglycerin into arterial grafts as well as the native coronary artery through cardiac catheter may relieve spasm and this could a life-saving procedure [54]. The method is used successfully by others to relieve the coronary spasm as well [170]. Due to the fact that radial artery spasm is a frequent complication of the transradial approach for coronary angiography and angioplasty, this method is now used in catheterization laboratory. Administration of an intra-arterial vasodilating cocktail composed of verapamil plus nitroglycerine prior to sheath insertion reduces the occurrence and severity of radial artery spasm [171].

IV.12. Balloon Calibration to Relieve IMA Spasm

This technique allows full IMA distention without the devascularizing effects of full skeletonization and was applied in more than 793 patients over five years. Postcalibration flow rates increased 3- to 18-fold over precalibration flow rates [200].

IV.13. Adenoviral Transfer of NOS

Adenoviral transfer of NOS suggests that future clinical application of gene therapy may play an important role in prevention of RA vasospasm [38].

IV.14. Extracorporeal Membrane Oxygenation (ECMO)

For diffuse refractory vascular spasm after CABG, a rare but lethal condition, an aggressive treatment, that is, prompt ECMO institution and controlled cardiocirculatory assistance, represents the preferred solution to face such a dramatic event and may save patient lives [59].

The above pharmacological and non-pharmacological antispastic methods have been summarized with detailed illustrations and tables in the two most recent review articles [201,202].

SUMMARY AND CONCLUSION

CABG surgery has been the standard treatment for patients with coronary artery disease particularly for three-vessel disease, although PCI has become the preferred method in one- or two-vessel disease. Arterial grafting using autologous arteries as the grafts has been demonstrated to have superior long-term results. Use of the left IMA to graft the diseased LAD has become the standard method for almost all CABG surgery and bilateral IMA grafts may further enhance survival over the long-term. Other arteries such as radial artery, right gastroepiploic artery, and inferior epigastric artery are commonly used arterial grafts. However, in comparison to vein grafts, arterial grafts have a tendency to develop vasospasm that can lead to potentially life-threatening complications. This is a long-recognized clinical problem and occurs even in the current practice. There have been various antispastic protocols, either pharmacological or non-pharmacological, but the rationale and efficacy are sometimes unclear. The multiple methods used in CABG to prevent and treat spasm of arterial grafts are effective in the current practice but it is still controversial as to what is the most effective regimen. This is partially due to the pathophysiological complexity of the mechanism of vascular spasm and the evolution of pharmacological vasodilators and non-pharmacological methods. Better understanding of the mechanism of vascular spasm, development of new pharmacological vasodilators, and the adequate evaluation of non-pharmacological methods may lead to a more unanimous opinion as to the best method to prevent and treat arterial spasm in contemporary clinical practice.

Funding Sources

The work described in this paper was fully supported by grants from the National Natural Science Foundation of China (81170148), Zhejiang Provincial Natural Science Foundation (LY15H020008), Hangzhou Science and Technology Projects (20140633B12), & Tianjin Binhai Key Platform for Creative Research Program (2012-BH110004), Binhai New Area Health Bureau (2012BWKZ 008, 2014BWKY002), Tianjin Health Bureau (2013KZ009).

Disclosures

None.

References

[1] Loop FD, Lytle BW, Cosgrove DM, Stewart RW, Goormastic M, Williams GW, Golding LA, Gill CC, Taylor PC, Sheldon WC. Influence of the internal- mammary-artery graft on 10-year survival and other cardiac events. *N Engl J Med* 1986; 314:1-6.

[2] Taggart DP. CABG or stents in coronary artery disease: end of the debate? *Lancet.* 2013 Feb 23;381:605-7.

[3] Sabik JF 3rd, Stockins A, Nowicki ER, Blackstone EH, Houghtaling PL, Lytle BW, Loop FD. Does location of the second internal thoracic artery graft influence outcome of coronary artery bypass grafting? *Circulation.* 2008;118:S210-5.

[4] Leacche M, Gosev I. Hybrid coronary revascularization: the future of coronary artery bypass surgery or an unfulfilled promise? *Circulation.* 2014 Jul 23. pii: CIRCULATION AHA.114.011857.

[5] Yi G, Shine B, Rehman SM, Altman DG, Taggart DP. Effect of bilateral internal mammary artery on long-term survival: a meta-analysis approach. *Circulation.* 2014 Jun 10. pii: CIRCULATION AHA.113.004255.

[6] Acar C, Jebara VA, Portoghese M, et al.: Revival of the radial artery for coronary bypass grafting. *Ann Thorac Surg* 1992;54:652-60.

[7] Rehman SM, Yi G, Taggart DP. The radial artery: current concepts on its use in coronary artery revascularization. *Ann Thorac Surg.* 2013;96:1900-9.

[8] Pym J, Brown PM, Charrette EJP, Parker JO, West RO. Gastroepiploic-coronary anastomosis: a viable alternative bypass graft. *J Thorac Cardiovasc Surg* 1987;94:256-9.

[9] Suma H, Wanibuchi Y, Furuta S, Isshiki T, Yamaguchi T, Takanashi R. Comparative study between the gastroepiploic and the internal thoracic artery as a coronary bypass graft. Size, flow, patency, histology. *Eur J Cardiothorac Surg.* 1991;5:244-7.

[10] Yokoyama Y, Matsushita S, Iesaki T, Yamamoto T, Inaba H, Okada T, Amano A. Denervation of gastroepiploic artery graft can reduce vasospasm. *J Thorac Cardiovasc Surg.* 2014;147:951-5.

[11] Puig LB, Ciongolli W, Cividanes GV, Dontos A, Kopel L, Bittencourt D, Assis RV, Jatene AD. Inferior epigastric artery as a free graft for myocardial revascularization. *J Thorac Cardiovasc Surg* 1990;99:251-5.

[12] Buche M, Schoevaerdts JC, Louagie Y, Schroeder E, Marchandise B, Chenu P, Dion R, Verhelst R, Deloos M, Gonzales E. Use of the inferior epigastric artery for coronary bypass. *J Thorac Cardiovasc Surg* 1992;103:665-70.

[13] Cunningham JN: Papaverine hydrochloride preservation of vein grafts. *J Thorac Cardiovasc Surg* 1982; 84:933-4.

[14] He GW, Rosenfeldt FL, Angus JA. Pharmacological relaxation of the saphenous vein during harvesting for coronary artery bypass grafting. *Ann Thorac Surg.* 1993;55:1210-7.

[15] He GW, Angus JA, Rosenfeldt FL: Reactivity of the canine isolated internal mammary artery, saphenous vein, and coronary artery to constrictor and dilator substances: Relevance to coronary bypass graft surgery. *J Cardiovasc Pharmacol* 1988;12:12-22.

[16] Luscher TF, Diederich D, Siebenmann R, et al. Difference between endothlium-dependent relaxation in arterial and in venous coronary bypass grafts. *N Engl J Med* 1988;319:462-7.

[17] He GW, Rosenfeldt F, Buxton B, Angus JA: Reactivity of human isolated internal mammary artery to constrictor and dilator agents. Implications for treatment of internal mammary artery spasm. *Circulation* 1989;80:I-141-50.

[18] Jett GK, Guyton RA, Hatcher CR, Abel PW: Inhibition of human internal mammary artery contractions. An in vitro study of vasodilators. *J Thorac Cardiovasc Surg* 1992;104:977-82.

[19] He GW, Shaw J, Yang CQ, et al. Inhibitory effects of glyceryl trinitrate on α-adrenoceptor mediated contraction in the internal mammary artery. *Br J Clin Pharmacol* 1992;34:236-43.
[20] Cooper GJ, Wilkinson GAL, Angilini GD: Overcoming perioperative spasm of the internal mammary artery: which is the best vasodilator? *J Thorac Cardiovasc Surg* 1992;104:465-8.
[21] He GW, Shaw J, Hughes C.F, et al. Predominant α1-adrenoceptor mediated contraction in the human internal mammary artery. *J Cardiovasc Pharmacol* 1993;21:256-63.
[22] Tatoulis J, Buxton BF, Fuller JA. Patencies of 2127 arterial to coronary conduits over 15 years. *Ann Thorac Surg*. 2004;77:93-101.
[23] He GW, Rosenfeldt FL, Angus JA, and Buxton, BF: Pharmacological dilatation of internal mammary artery during surgery. J *Thorac Cardiovasc Surg* 1994;107:1440-4.
[24] Cooper GJ, Locke TJ: The in vitro response of human internal mammary artery to vasodilators. *J Thorac Cadiovasc Surg* 1994;107:1155-6.
[25] Dietle CA, Benoit CH: Radial artery graft for coronary revascularization: Technical considerations. *Ann Thorac Surg* 1995;60:102-10.
[26] Seo B, Oemar BS, Siebenmann R, von Segesser L, Luscher TF: Both ETA and ETB receptors mediate contraction to endothelin-1 in human blood vessels. *Circulation* 1994;89:1203-8.
[27] Reyes AT, Frame R, Brodman RF. Technique for harvesting the radial artery as a coronary artery bypass graft. *Ann Thorac Surg* 1995;59:118-26.
[28] Esmore DS, Burton PR, Smith JA, Rabinov M, Pick A, McMahon J, Rosenfeldt FL. A simplified method of harvesting and dilating the radial artery achieves acceptable clinical outcomes. *Aust N Z J Surg. 2000*;70:366-70.
[29] He GW, Yang CQ: Comparison among arterial grafts and coronary artery. An attempt at functional classification. *J Thorac Cardiovasc Surg* 1995;109:707-15.
[30] He GW, Acuff TE, Yang CQ, Ryan WH, Mack MJ: Functional comparison between the human inferior epigastric artery and internal mammary artery: Similarities and differences. *J Thorac Cardiovasc Surg* 1995;109:13-20.
[31] He GW, Yang CQ: Effects of thromboxane A2 antagonist GR32191B on prostanoid and nonprostanoid receptors in the human internal mammary artery. *J Cardiovasc Pharmacol* 1995;26:13-9.

[32] Kiessling AH, Romasku D, Beiras-Fernandez A, Ferreirós N, Labocha S, Moritz A, Rastan AJ. Pharmacokinetics of intraluminally administered serum papaverine for spasm prophylaxis of the internal mammary artery. *Heart Surg Forum.* 2013;16:E266-70.

[33] He GW, Yang CQ, Gately H, et al: Potential greater than additive vasorelaxant actions of milrinone and nitroglycerin on human conduit arteries. *Br J Clin Pharmacol* 1996;41:101-7.

[34] He GW, Yang CQ: Use of verapamil and nitroglycerin solution in preparation of radial artery for coronary grafting. *Ann Thorac Surg* 1996;61:610-4.

[35] He GW, Yang CQ: Comparison of nitroprusside and nitroglycerin in inhibition of angiotensin II and other vasoconstrictor-mediated contraction in human coronary bypass conduits. *Br J Clin Pharmacol* 1997;44:361-7.

[36] He GW: Verapamil plus nitroglycerin solution maximally preserves endothelial function of the radial artery: comparison to papaverine solution. *J Thorac Cardiovasc Surg* 1998;115:1321-7.

[37] He GW, Yang CQ: Characteristics of adrenoceptors in the human radial artery: clinical implications. *J Thorac Cardiovasc Surg* 1998;115:1136-41.

[38] Cable DG, Caccitolo JA, Pearson PJ, O'Brien T, Mullany CJ, Daly RC, Orszulak TA, Schaff HV: New approaches to prevention and treatment of radial artery graft vasospasm. *Circulation* 1998; 98:II15-21; discussion II21-2.

[39] Rosenfeldt FL, He GW, Buxton BF, Angus JA: Pharmacology of coronary artery bypass grafts. *Ann Thorac Surg* 1999;67:878-88.

[40] Chavanon O, Cracowski JL, Hacini R, Stanke F, Durand M, Noirclerc M, Blin D: Effect of topical vasodilators on gastroepiploic artery graft. *Ann Thorac Surg* 1999;67:1295-8.

[41] He GW, Yang CQ: Comparison of vasorelaxant effect of nitroprusside and nitroglycerin in the human radial artery. *Br J Clin Pharmacol* 1999;48:99-104.

[42] Shapira OM, Xu A, Vita JA, Aldea GS, Shah N, Shemin RJ, Keaney JF Jr: Nitroglycerin is superior to diltiazem as a coronary bypass conduit vasodilator. *J Thorac Cardiovasc Surg* 1999;117:906-11.

[43] He GW, Yang CQ: Comparative study on calcium channel antagonists in the human radial artery: clinical implications. *J Thorac Cardiovasc Surg* 2000;119:94-100.

[44] Zabeeda D, Medalion B, Jackobshvilli S, Ezra S, Schachner A, Cohen AJ: Comparison of systemic vasodilators: effects on flow in internal mammary and radial arteries. *Ann Thorac Surg* 2001;71:138-41.

[45] Gabe ED, Figal JC, Wisner JN, Laguens R: Radial artery graft vasospasm. *Eur J Cardiothorac Surg* 2001;19:102-4.

[46] Lobato EB, Janelle GM, Urdaneta F, Martin TD: Comparison of milrinone versus nitroglycerin, alone and in combination, on grafted internal mammary artery flow after cardiopulmonary bypass: effects of alpha-adrenergic stimulation. *J Cardiothorac Vasc Anesth* 2001;15:723-7.

[47] Wei W, H. Storm Floten, He GW: Interaction between vasodilators and vasopressin in internal mammary artery and clinical significance. *Ann Thorac Surg* 2002;73:516-22.

[48] Sarabu MR, McClung JA, Fass A, Reed GE. Early postoperative spasm in left internal mammary artery bypass grafts. *Ann Thorac Surg.* 1987;44:199-200.

[49] Hata M, Shiono M, Orime Y, Hata H, Yagi S, Tsukamoto S, Kimura S, Sezai A, Kashiwawzaki S, Choh S, Negishi N, Sezai Y. Spontaneous recanalization of postoperative severe graft stenosis. What is the cause and prognosis of the "string sign" in the internal thoracic artery? *Ann Thorac Cardiovasc Surg.* 1999;5:52-5.

[50] Jones EL, Lattouf OM, Weintraub WS. Catastrophic consequences of internal mammary artery hypoperfusion. *J Thorac Cardiovasc Surg.* 1989;98:902-7.

[51] Fakiolas CN1, Adamopoulou EN, Kouvaras GA, Olympios CD, Foussas SG. Systolic segmental disappearance of internal mammary artery graft. Correlation with prolonged spasm of the graft. *Acta Cardiol.* 1995;50(1):71-7.

[52] He GW. Contractility of the human internal mammary artery at the distal section increases toward the end. Emphasis on not using the end of the internal mammary artery for grafting. *J Thorac Cardiovasc Surg.* 1993;106:406-11.

[53] Vogt PR, Hess O, Turina MI. Internal mammary artery spasm immediately after grafting to the left anterior descending artery: diagnosis and treatment. *Eur Heart J.* 1996;17:804.

[54] He GW, Fan KY, Chiu SW, Chow WH. Injection of vasodilators into arterial grafts through cardiac catheter to relieve spasm. *Ann Thorac Surg.* 2000;69:625-8.

[55] Sanders LH, Newman MA. Intractable postoperative internal thoracic artery spasm managed with angiographic intraluminal papaverine. *J Thorac Cardiovasc Surg*. 2005;130:938-40.

[56] Harskamp RE, McNeil JD, van Ginkel MW, Bastos RB, Baisden CE, Calhoon JH. Postoperative internal thoracic artery spasm after coronary artery bypass grafting. *Ann Thorac Surg*. 2008;85:647-9.

[57] Pratt GF, Erickson M, Provenzano S, Mews G, Edwards M. Intractable LIMA spasm in the postoperative period treated by placement of 'bridging' stent. *Ann Thorac Surg*. 2008;86:1985-7.

[58] Baek JH1, Han SS, Lee DH. Native coronary artery and grafted artery spasm just after coronary artery bypass grafting: a case report. *J Korean Med Sci*. 2010 ;25:641-3.

[59] Lorusso R, Crudeli E, Lucà F, De Cicco G, Vizzardi E, D'Aloia A, Gelsomino S. Refractory spasm of coronary arteries and grafted conduits after isolated coronary artery bypass surgery. *Ann Thorac Surg*. 2012;93:545-51.

[60] Nakazawa H, Moriyama K, Motoyasu A, Endo H, Kubota H, Yorozu T. Prompt institution of percutaneous cardiopulmonary support managed perioperative refractory vascular spasm after isolated coronary artery bypass grafting surgery. *Gen Thorac Cardiovasc Surg*. 2013;61:711-5.

[61] Ichikawa Y1, Kajiwara H, Hamada T, Yamazaki I, Jin Y, Sato S. Late vasospasm of the inferior epigastric artery graft. *Ann Thorac Surg*. 1999;67:1800-1.

[62] He GW. Arterial grafts for coronary artery bypass grafting: biological characteristics, functional classification, and clinical choice. *Ann Thorac Surg*. 1999;67:277-84.

[63] Liu ZG, Ge ZD, He GW. Difference in endothelium-derived hyperpolarizing factor-mediated hyperpolarization and nitric oxide release between human internal mammary artery and saphenous vein. *Circulation*. 2000;102:III296-301.

[64] He GW, Liu ZG. Comparison of nitric oxide release and endothelium-derived hyperpolarizing factor-mediated hyperpolarization between human radial and internal mammary arteries. *Circulation*. 2001;104:I344-9.

[65] He GW, Yang CQ. Radial artery has higher receptor-mediated contractility but similar endothelial function compared with mammary artery. *Ann Thorac Surg* 1997;63:1346-52.

[66] He GW, Fan L, Grove KL, Furnary A, Yang Q. Expression and function of endothelial nitric oxide synthase messenger RNA and protein are

higher in internal mammary than in radial arteries. *Ann Thorac Surg.* 2011;92:845-50.

[67] Choudhary BP, Antoniades C, Brading AF, Galione A, Channon K, Taggart DP. Diabetes mellitus as a predictor for radial artery vasoreactivity in patients undergoing coronary artery bypass grafting. *J Am Coll Cardiol.* 2007;50:1047-53.

[68] Yaqub Y, Suarez J, Perez-Verdia A, Arvandi A, Nugent KM. Klippel-Trenaunay syndrome and radial artery coronary graft spasm. *J Coll Physicians Surg Pak.* 2009;19:658-60.

[69] Kulkarni NM, Thomas MR. Severe spasm of a radial artery coronary bypass graft during coronary intervention. *Catheter Cardiovasc Interv.* 1999;47:331-5.

[70] Gabe ED, Figal JC, Wisner JN, Laguens R. Radial artery graft vasospasm. *Eur J Cardiothorac Surg.* 2001;19:102-4.

[71] Goube P, Hammoudi N, Pagny JY, Boutekadjirt R, Toledano D, Achouh P, Acar C. Radial artery graft stenosis treated by percutaneous intervention. *Eur J Cardiothorac Surg.* 2010;37:697-703.

[72] Suma H. Spasm of the gastroepiploic artery graft. *Ann Thorac Surg* 1990;49:168-9.

[73] Mills NL, Hockmuth DR, Everson CT, Robart CC. Right gastroepiploic artery used for coronary artery bypass grafting. Evaluation of flow characteristics and size. *J Thorac Cardiovasc Surg.* 1993;106:579-85.

[74] Cate CM, Gitter R, Jett K. Spasm of the gastroepiploic artery used for coronary artery bypass grafting. *Am J Cardiol.* 1996 ;77:1022-3.

[75] Hara K, Kashida M, Tamura T, Saeki F, Ikari Y, Suma H. Diffuse spasm of a free gastroepiploic artery graft during percutaneous balloon angioplasty. *Cathet Cardiovasc Diagn.* 1994;33:136-8.

[76] Van Son JAM, Smedts F, Vincent JG, Van Lier HJ, Kubat K. Comparative anatomic studies of various arterial conduits for myocardial revascularization. *J Thorac Cardiovasc Surg* 1990;99:703-7.

[77] He GW, Yang CQ, Starr A: An overview of the nature of vasoconstriction in arterial grafts for coronary surgery. *Ann Thorac Surg* 1995;59:676-83.

[78] Lockowandt U, Ritchie A, Grossebener M, Franco-Cereceda A. Endothelin and effects of endothelin-receptor activation in the mammary and radial artery. *Scand Cardiovasc J.* 2004;38:240-4.

[79] Cross KS, el-Sanadiki MN, Murray JJ, Mikat EM, McCann RL, Hagen PO. Mast cell infiltration: a possible mechanism for vein graft vasospasm. *Surgery.* 1988;104:171-7.

[80] He GW, Buxton B, Rosenfeldt FL, Wilson AC, Angus JA. Weak beta-adrenoceptor-mediated relaxation in the human internal mammary artery. *J Thorac Cardiovasc Surg.* 1989;97:259-66.
[81] Kitamura S1, Morita R, Kawachi K, Iioka S, Seki T, Inoue K, Taniguchi S. Different responses of coronary artery and internal mammary artery bypass grafts to ergonovine and nitroglycerin in variant angina. *Ann Thorac Surg.* 1989;47:756-60.
[82] Wei W, Yang CQ, Furnary A, He GW: Greater vasopressin-induced vasoconstriction and inferior effects of nitrovasodilators and milrinone in the radial artery than in the internal thoracic artery. *J Thorac Cardiovasc Surg* 2005;129:33-40.
[83] Stojnic N, Bukarica LG, Peric M, Bumbasirevic M, Lesic A, Lipkovski JM, Heinle H. Analysis of vasoreactivity of isolated human radial artery. *J Pharmacol Sci.* 2006;100:34-40.
[84] Arshad M, Vijay V, Floyd BC, Marks B, Sarabu MR, Wolin MS, Gupte SA. Thromboxane receptor stimulation suppresses guanylate cyclase-mediated relaxation of radial arteries. *Ann Thorac Surg.* 2006;81:2147-54.
[85] Liu JJ, Chen JR, Bradley CJ, Xie B, Johnston CI, Buxton BF. Autologous neutrophil derived supernatants inhibit endothelium dependent relaxation in human coronary bypass graft. *Cardiovasc Res.* 1994 ;28:1353-9.
[86] Kun X, Lefeng W, Rongjing D, Xincun Y. RhoA/ROK pathway related to the mechanism of higher susceptibility to spasm in RA than in IMA. *J Card Surg.* 2009;24:766-71.
[87] Mueed I, Tazzeo T, Liu C, Pertens E, Zhang Y, Cybulski I, Semelhago L, Noora J, Lamy A, Teoh K, Chu V, Janssen LJ. Isoprostanes constrict human radial artery by stimulation of thromboxane receptors, $Ca2^+$ release, and RhoA activation. *J Thorac Cardiovasc Surg.* 2008;135: 131-8.
[88] Aghamohammadzadeh R, Withers S, Lynch F, Greenstein A, Malik R, Heagerty A. Perivascular adipose tissue from human systemic and coronary vessels: the emergence of a new pharmacotherapeutic target. *Br J Pharmacol.* 2012;165:670-82.
[89] Bodelsson M, Arneklo-Nobin B, Chester AH, Tadjkarimi S, Törnebrandt K, Yacoub M. Differential effect of hypothermia on the vascular tone and reactivity of the human coronary artery and graft vessels. *J Cardiovasc Surg (Torino).* 1991 ;32:288-94.

[90] Chen Z, Zhang J, Stamler JS. Identification of the enzymatic mechanism of nitroglycerin bioactivation. *Proc Natl Acad Sci U S A*. 2002;99:8306-11.

[91] Mills NL, Bringaze WL 3rd.Preparation of the internal mammary artery graft. Which is the best method? *J Thorac Cardiovasc Surg*. 1989;98:73-7; discussion 78-9.

[92] Martin W, Furchgott RF, Villani GM, Jothianandan: Phosphodiesterase inhibitors induce endothelium-dependent relaxation of rat and rabbit aorta by potentiating the effects of spontaneously released endothelium-derived relaxing factor. *J Pharmacol Exp Ther* 1986;237:539-47.

[93] Fujioka M. Lack of a causal relationship between the vasodilator effect of papaverine and cyclic AMP production in the dog basilar artery. *Br J Pharmoc* 1984;83:113-24.

[94] Brading AF, Burdyga TV, Scripnyuk ZD. The effects of papaverine on the electrical and mechanical activity of the guinea-pig ureter. *J Physiol* 1983;334:79-89.

[95] Dregelid E, Heldal K, Resch F, Stangeland L, Breivik K, Svendsen E. Dilation of the internal mammary artery by external and intraluminal papaverine application. *J Thorac Cardiovasc Surg*. 1995;110:697-703.

[96] Sasson L, Cohen AJ, Hauptman E, Schachner A. Effect of topical vasodilators on internal mammary arteries. *Ann Thorac Surg*. 1995;59:494-6.

[97] Bilgen F, Yapici MF, Serbetçioğlu A, Tarhan IA, Coruh T, Ozler A. Effect of normothermic papaverine to relieve intraoperative spasm of the internal thoracic artery. *Ann Thorac Surg*. 1996;62:769-71.

[98] Yavuz S, Celkan A, Göncü T, Türk T, Ozdemir IA. Effect of papaverine applications on blood flow of the internal mammary artery. *Ann Thorac Cardiovasc Surg*. 2001;7:84-8.

[99] Girard DS, Sutton JP 3rd, Williams TH, Crumbley AJ 3rd, Zellner JL, Kratz JM, Crawford FA. Papaverine delivery to the internal mammary artery pedicle effectively treats spasm. *Ann Thorac Surg*. 2004;78: 1295-8.

[100] Bahcivan M, Kolbakir F, Karamustafa H, Keceligil HT. Endothoracic papaverine application for internal thoracic artery harvest. *Asian Cardiovasc Thorac Ann*. 2007;15:234-7.

[101] Suma H, Wanibuchi Y, Furuta S, Isshiki T, Yamaguchi T, Takanashi R. Comparative study between the gastroepiploic and the internal thoracic artery as a coronary bypass graft. Size, flow, patency, histology. *Eur J Cardiothorac Surg*. 1991;5:244-7.

[102] Chavanon O, Cracowski JL, Hacini R, Stanke F, Durand M, Noirclerc M, Blin D. Effect of topical vasodilators on gastroepiploic artery graft. *Ann Thorac Surg.* 1999;67:1295-8.

[103] Ignarro LJ. After 130 years, the molecular mechanism of action of nitroglycerin is revealed. *Proc Natl Acad Sci U S A.* 2002; 99: 7816–7817.

[104] Jett GK, Arcici JM Jr, Hatcher CR Jr, Abel PW, Guyton RA. Vasodilator drug effects on internal mammary artery and saphenous vein grafts. *J Am Coll Cardiol.* 1988;11:1317-24.

[105] Uydeş-Doğan BS, Nebigil M, Aslamaci S, Onuk E, Kanzik I, Akar F. The comparison of vascular reactivities of arterial and venous grafts to vasodilators: management of graft spasm. *Int J Cardiol.* 1996;53:137-45.

[106] Gurevitch J, Miller HI, Shapira I, Kramer A, Paz Y, Matsa M, Mohr R, Yakirevich V. High-dose isosorbide dinitrate for myocardial revascularization with composite arterial grafts. *Ann Thorac Surg.* 1997;63:382-7.

[107] Shapira OM, Alkon JD, Macron DS, Keaney JF Jr, Vita JA, Aldea GS, Shemin RJ. Nitroglycerin is preferable to diltiazem for prevention of coronary bypass conduit spasm. *Ann Thorac Surg.* 2000 ;70:883-8; discussion 888-9.

[108] Ding R, Feng W, Li H, Wang L, Li D, Cheng Z, Guo J, Hu D. A comparative study on in vitro and in vivo effects of topical vasodilators in human internal mammary, radial artery and great saphenous vein. *Eur J Cardiothorac Surg.* 2008;34:536-41.

[109] Kiss L, Benko R, Kovács E, Szerafin T, Módis K, Szabó C, Lacza Z. Human internal thoracic artery grafts exhibit severe morphological and functional damage and spasmic vasomotion due to oxidative stress. *Med Sci Monit.* 2011;17:CR411-6.

[110] Nisanoglu V, Battaloglu B, Ozgur B, Eroglu T, Erdil N. Topical vasodilators for preventing radial artery spasm during harvesting for coronary revascularization: comparison of 4 agents. *Heart Surg Forum.* 2006;9:E807-12.

[111] Sogo N, Campanella C, Webb DJ, Megson IL. S-nitrosothiols cause prolonged, nitric oxide-mediated relaxation in human saphenous vein and internal mammary artery: therapeutic potential in bypass surgery. *Br J Pharmacol.* 2000;131:1236-44.

[112] Liu JJ, Johnston CI, Buxton BF: Synergistic effect of nisoldipine and nitroglycerin on human internal mammary artery. *J Pharmacol Exp Therap* 1994;268:434-40.

[113] Chanda J, Canver CC. Reversal of preexisting vasospasm in coronary artery conduits. *Ann Thorac Surg*. 2001;72:476-80.
[114] He GW, Fan L, Furnary A, Yang Q. A new antispastic solution for arterial grafting: nicardipine and nitroglycerin cocktail in preparation of internal thoracic and radial arteries for coronary surgery. *J Thorac Cardiovasc Surg*. 2008;136:673-80, 680.e1-2.
[115] Zheng SY, Wu M, Huang JS, Mai MJ, Chen TB, He GW. Use of antispastic nicardipine and nitroglycerin (NG) cocktail solution increases graft flow during off-pump coronary artery bypass grafting. *J Cardiovasc Surg (Torino)*. 2012;53:783-8.
[116] He GW. Aterial grafts: clinical classification and pharmacological management. *Ann Cardiothorac Surg*. 2013 Jul;2(4):507-18.
[117] Bai XY, Liu XC, Jing WB, Yang Q, Tang XD, He GW. Effect of amlodipine in human internal mammary artery and clinical implications. *Ann Thorac Surg*. 2010;90:1952-7.
[118] Fan L, Yang Q, Xiao XQ, Grove KL, Huang Y, Chen ZW, Furnary A, He GW. Dual actions of cilnidipine in human internal thoracic artery: inhibition of calcium channels and enhancement of endothelial nitric oxide synthase. *J Thorac Cardiovasc Surg*. 2011;141:1063-9.
[119] Gao G, Liu XC, Jing WB, Yang Q, He GW. Vasorelaxation induced by new third-generation dihydropyridine calcium antagonist azelnidipine in human internal mammary artery. *Ann Thorac Surg*. 2013;96:1316-21.
[120] Tabel Y, Hepağuşlar H, Erdal C, Catalyürek H, Acikel U, Elar Z, Aslan O. Diltiazem provides higher internal mammary artery flow than nitroglycerin during coronary artery bypass grafting surgery. *Eur J Cardiothorac Surg*. 2004;25:553-9.
[121] Chanda J, Brichkov I, Canver CC. Prevention of radial artery graft vasospasm after coronary bypass. *Ann Thorac Surg*. 2000;70:2070-4.
[122] He GW, Acuff TE, Ryan WH, Yang CQ, Douthit MB, Bowman RT, Mack MJ. Inhibitory effects of calcium antagonists on alpha-adrenoceptor-mediated contraction in the human internal mammary artery. *Br J Clin Pharmacol*. 1994;37:173-9.
[123] He GW, Yang CQ, Mack MJ, Acuff TE, Ryan WH, Starr A. Interaction between endothelin and vasodilators in the human internal mammary artery. *Br J Clin Pharmacol*. 1994;38:505-12.
[124] Wei W, Floten HS, He GW: Interaction between vasodilators and vasopressin in internal mammary artery and clinical significance. *Ann Thorac Surg* 2002;73:516-22.

[125] Beavo JA, Reifsnyder DH: Primary sequences of cyclic nucleotide phosphodiesterases isozymes and the design of selective inhibitors. *Trends Pharmacol Sci* 1990;11:150-5.
[126] He G-W and Yang C-Q: Inhibition of vasoconstriction by phosphodiesterase III inhibitor milrinone in human conduit arteries used as coronary bypass grafts. *J Cardiovasc Pharmacol* 1996;28:208-14.
[127] Liu JJ, Doolan LA, Xie B, Chen JR, Buxton BF. Direct vasodilator effect of milrinone, an inotropic dgug, on arterial coronary bypass grafts. *J Thorac Cardiovasc Surg* 1997;113:3108-13.
[128] García-Rinaldi R, Soltero ER, Carballido J, Mojica J. Intraluminal milrinone for dilation of the radial artery graft. *Tex Heart Inst J.* 1999;26:189-91.
[129] He GW, Yang CQ: Vasorelaxant effect of phosphodiesterase-inhibitor milrinone in the human radial artery used as coronary bypass graft. *J Thorac Cardiovasc Surg* 2000;119:1039-45.
[130] Yamaguchi S, Watanabe G, Higasidani K, Tomita S, Iino K, Ujiie T, Yamamoto S. Skeletonized radial artery graft prepared with phosphodiesterase-III inhibitors indicates favorable results compared with pedicled radial artery graft in angiographic studies. *Innovations* (Phila). 2006;1:251-4.
[131] Lobato EB, Janelle GM, Urdaneta F, Martin TD: Comparison of milrinone versus nitroglycerin, alone and in combination, on grafted internal mammary artery flow after cardiopulmonary bypass: effects of alpha-adrenergic stimulation. *J Cardiothorac Vasc Anesth* 2001;15: 723-7.
[132] Möllhoff T, Schmidt C, Van Aken H, Berendes E, Buerkle H, Marmann P, Reinbold T, Prenger-Berninghoff R, Tjan TD, Scheld HH, Deng MC. Myocardial ischaemia in patients with impaired left ventricular function undergoing coronary artery bypass grafting--milrinone versus nifedipin. *Eur J Anaesthesiol.* 2002;19:796-802.
[133] Cracowski JL, Stanke-Labesque F, Chavanon O, Blin D, Mallion JM, Bessard G, Devillier P: Vasorelaxant actions of enoximone, dobutamine, and the combination on human arterial coronary bypass grafts. *J Cardiovasc Pharmacol* 1999;34:741-8.
[134] Yan M, Liu DL, Chua YL, Chen C, Lim YL. Tyrosine kinase inhibitors suppress alpha1-adrenoceptor mediated contraction in human radial, internal mammary arteries and saphenous vein. *Neurosci Lett.* 2002;333:171-4.

[135] Mussa S, Guzik TJ, Black E, Dipp MA, Channon KM, Taggart DP. Comparative efficacies and durations of action of phenoxybenzamine, verapamil/nitroglycerin solution, and papaverine as topical antispasmodics for radial artery coronary bypass grafting. *J Thorac Cardiovasc Surg* 2003;126:1798-805.

[136] Corvera JS, Morris CD, Budde JM, Velez DA, Puskas JD, Lattouf OM, Cooper WA, Guyton RA, Vinten-Johansen J. Pretreatment with phenoxybenzamine attenuates the radial artery's vasoconstrictor response to alpha-adrenergic stimuli. *J Thorac Cardiovasc Surg* 2003;126:1549-54.

[137] Dipp MA, Nye PC, Taggart DP. Phenoxybenzamine is more effective and less harmful than papaverine in the prevention of radial artery vasospasm. *Eur J Cardiothorac Surg.* 2001;19:482-6.

[138] Harrison WE, Mellor AJ, Clark J, Singer DR. Vasodilator pre-treatment of human radial arteries; comparison of effects of phenoxybenzamine vs papaverine on norepinephrine-induced contraction in vitro. *Eur Heart J.* 2001;22:2209-16.

[139] Conant AR, Shackcloth MJ, Oo AY, Chester MR, Simpson AW, Dihmis WC: Phenoxybenzamine treatment is insufficient to prevent spasm in the radial artery: the effect of other vasodilators. *J Thorac Cardiovasc Surg* 2003;126:448-54.

[140] Liu MH, Floten HS, Yang Q, He GW. Inhibition of vasoconstriction by AJ-2615, a novel calcium antagonist with α1-adrenergic receptor blocking activity in human conduit arteries used as bypass grafts. *Br J Clin Pharmacol* 2001;52:279-87.

[141] Shafiei M, Omrani G, Mahmoudian M: Coexistence of at least three distinct beta-adrenoceptors in human internal mammary artery. *Acta Physiol Hung* 2000;87:275-86.

[142] Katai R, Tsuneyoshi I, Hamasaki J, Onomoto M, Suehiro S, Sakata R, Kanmura Y: The variable effects of dopamine among human isolated arteries commonly used for coronary bypass grafts. *Anesth Analg* 2004;98:915-20.

[143] Halpenny M, Lakshmi S, O'Donnell A, O'Callaghan-Enright S, O'Connell D, Shorten G. The effects of fenoldopam on coronary conduit blood flow after coronary artery bypass graft surgery. *J Cardiothorac Vasc Anesth.* 2001;15:72-6.

[144] Ozdemir C, Ikizler M, Besogul Y, Karakaya A, Sirmagul B. An alternative agent for radial arterial graft spasm: application of topical iloprost. *Scand Cardiovasc J.* 2007;41:201-6.

[145] Ege T, Gur O, Karadag CH, Duran E. Evaluation of iloprost to prevent vasospasm in coronary artery bypass grafts. *J Int Med Res.* 2010;38:1759-63.

[146] Ustunsoy H, Kazaz H, Celkan MA, Deniz H, Davutoglu V, Bakir K, Cine N, Burma O. Randomized comparison of vasodilator effects of iloprost versus diltiazem on flow and pathologic changes in radial arteries: mid-term angiographic control study of the comparison of vasodilators on radial artery vasospasm. *Heart Surg Forum.* 2009;12:E202-7.

[147] Kun X, Lefeng W, Rongjing D, Xincun Y. RhoA/ROK pathway related to the mechanism of higher susceptibility to spasm in RA than in IMA. *J Card Surg.* 2009;24:766-71.

[148] Inokuchi K, Ito A, Fukumoto Y, Matoba T, Shiose A, Nishida T, Masuda M, Morita S, Shimokawa H. Usefulness of fasudil, a Rho-kinase inhibitor, to treat intractable severe coronary spasm after coronary artery bypass surgery. *J Cardiovasc Pharmacol.* 2004;44:275-7.

[149] Watanabe G, Yamaguchi S, Takagi T, Tomita S, Tuan PM. Potent Vasodilatory Effect of Fasudil on Radial Artery Graft in Coronary Artery Bypass Operations. *Ann Thorac Surg.* 2013. pii: S0003-4975(13)02341-2.

[150] Liu MH, Floten HS, Furnary A, He GW: Inhibition of vasoconstriction by angiotensin receptor antagonist GR117289C in arteries grafts. *Ann Thorac Surg* 2000;70:2064-9.

[151] Achouh P, Simonet S, Badier-Commander C, Chardigny C, Vayssettes-Courchay C, Zegdi R, Khabbaz Z, Fabiani JN, Verbeuren TJ. The induction of heme oxygenase 1 decreases contractility in human internal thoracic artery and radial artery grafts. *J Thorac Cardiovasc Surg.* 2005;130:1573-80.

[152] Kelsall CJ, Chester AH, Amrani M, Singer DR. C-type natriuretic peptide relaxes human coronary artery bypass grafts preconstricted by endothelin-1. *Ann Thorac Surg.* 2005;80:1347-51.

[153] He GW, Yang CQ. Effect of thromboxane A2 antagonist GR32191B on prostanoid and nonprostanoid receptors in the human internal mammary artery. *J Cardiovasc Pharmacol.* 1995;26:13-9.

[154] He GW, Yang CQ. Inhibition of vasoconstriction by thromboxane A2 antagonist GR32191B in the human radial artery. *Br J Clin Pharmacol* 1999;48:207-15.

[155] Liu MH, Jin HK, Floten HS, Ren Z, Yim APC, He GW: Vascular endothelial growth factor-mediated, endothelium-dependent relaxation in human internal mammary artery. *Ann Thorac Surg* 2002;73:819-24.

[156] Wei W, Jin H, Chen ZW, Zioncheck TF, Yim APC, He GW: Vascular endothelial growth factor-induced nitric oxide- and PGI2-dependent relaxation in human internal mammary arteries: a comparative study with KDR and Flt-1 selective mutants. *J Cardiovasc Pharmacol* 2004;44:615-21.

[157] Lazdunski M: ATP-sensitive potassium channels: an overview. *J Cardiovasc Pharmacol* 1994;24:S1-5.

[158] Atwal KS: Pharmacology and structure-active relationships for KATP modulators: tissue-selective KATP openers. *J Cardiovasc Pharmacol* 1994;24:S12-7.

[159] He GW and Yang CQ: Inhibition of vasoconstriction by potassium channel opener aprikalim in human conduit arteries. *Br J Clin Pharmacol* 1997;44:353-9.

[160] Liu MH, Floten HS, Furnary A, Yim APC, He GW: Effect of potassium channel opener (KCO) aprikalim on the receptor-mediated vasoconstriction in the human internal mammary artery (IMA). *Ann Thorac Surg* 2001;71:636-41.

[161] Akar F, Uydeş-Dogan BS, Tufan H, Aşlamaci S, Köksoy C, Kanzik I. The comparison of the responsiveness of human isolated internal mammary and gastroepiploic arteries to levcromakalim: an alternative approach to the management of graft spasm. *Br J Clin Pharmacol* 1997;44:49-56.

[162] Novaković A, Gojković-Bukarica L, Beleslin-Cokić B, Japundzić-Zigon N, Sajić Z, Nezić D, Perić M, Djukanović B, Kazić T. Differential antivasoconstrictor effects of levcromakalim and rilmakalim on the isolated human mammary artery and saphenous vein. *J Pharmacol Sci.* 2003;92:108-14.

[163] Ren Z, Floten HS, Furnary A, Liu MH, Gately H, Swanson J, Ahmad A, Yim APC, He GW: Effects of potassium channel opener KRN4884 on human conduit arteries used as coronary bypass grafts. *Br J Clin Pharmacol* 2000;50:154-60.

[164] Li XN, Stulz P, Siebenmann RP, Yang Z, Lüscher TF. Different effects of activated platelets in the right gastroepiploic and internal mammary arteries. Implications for coronary artery grafting. *J Thorac Cardiovasc Surg.* 1992;104:1294-302.

[165] Güçlü O, Yüksel V, Hüseyin S, Ege T, Canbaz S, Süngün M. In vitro effects of L-carnitine on coronary artery bypass grafts. *Exp Clin Cardiol.* 2013 Spring;18:118-20.

[166] Murakami E, Iwata H, Imaizumi M, Takemura H. Prevention of arterial graft spasm by botulinum toxin: an in-vitro experiment. *Interact Cardiovasc Thorac Surg.* 2009;9:395-8.

[167] Berkan O, Bagcivan I, Kaya T, Yildirim K, Yildirim S, Doğan K. Investigation of the vasorelaxant effects of 3-(5'-hydroxymethyl-2'-furyl)-1-benzyl indazole (YC-1) and diethylamine/nitric oxide (DEA/NO) on the human radial artery used as coronary bypass graft. *Can J Physiol Pharmacol.* 2007;85:521-6.

[168] Formica F, Ferro O, Brustia M, Corti F, Colagrande L, Bosisio E, Paolini G. Effects of papaverine and glycerylnitrate-verapamil solution as topical and intraluminal vasodilators for internal thoracic artery. *Ann Thorac Surg.* 2006 ;81:120-4.

[169] Yoshizaki T, Tabuchi N, Toyama M. Verapamil and nitroglycerin improves the patency rate of radial artery grafts. *Asian Cardiovasc Thorac Ann. 2008*;16:396-400.

[170] Caputo M, Nicolini F, Franciosi G, Gallotti R: Coronary artery spasm after coronary artery bypass grafting. *Eur J Cardiothorac Surg* 1999;15:545-8.

[171] Kiemeneij F, Vajifdar BU, Eccleshall SC, Laarman G, Slagboom T, van der Wieken R: Evaluation of a spasmolytic cocktail to prevent radial artery spasm during coronary procedures. *Catheter Cardiovasc Interv* 2003;58:281-4.

[172] Li R, Amano A, Miyagawa H, Dohi S, Hayashi I, Kajimoto K, Shimada A, Hirose H. Skeletonized gastroepiploic artery for off-pump coronary artery bypass grafting. *Heart Surg Forum.* 2004;7:E164-9.

[173] Asai T, Tabata S. Skeletonization of the right gastroepiploic artery using an ultrasonic scalpel. *Ann Thorac Surg.* 2002;74:1715-7.

[174] Amano A, Takahashi A, Hirose H. Skeletonized radial artery grafting: improved angiographic results. *Ann Thorac Surg.* 2002;73:1880-7.

[175] Hirose H, Amano A. Skeletonized radial artery grafting: one-year patency rate. *Heart Surg Forum.* 2004;7:E277-82.

[176] Kucukarslan N, Kirilmaz A, Sungun M, Ozal E, Ulusoy RE, Sanisoglu Y, Tatar H. Harvesting of the radial artery: subfasciotomy or full skeletonization: a comparative study. *J Card Surg.* 2008;23:341-5.

[177] Rukosujew A, Reichelt R, Fabricius AM, Drees G, Tjan TD, Rothenburger M, Hoffmeier A, Scheld HH, Schmid C. Skeletonization

versus pedicle preparation of the radial artery with and without the ultrasonic scalpel. *Ann Thorac Surg.* 2004;77:120-5.

[178] Matsuura A, Yasuura K, Yoshida K, Oshima H, Tomari S, Ishida H, Mori S, Fujii G, Iwata K. Transplantation of the en bloc vascular system for coronary revascularization. *J Thorac Cardiovasc Surg.* 2001;121:520-5.

[179] Eda T, Miyahara K, Oshima H, Usui A, Matsuura A, Ueda Y. En-bloc free gastroepiploic artery graft provides a good long-term patency rate. *Asian Cardiovasc Thorac Ann.* 2010;18:244-9.

[180] Ozkan M, Koramaz I, Ulus AT, Tavil Y, Filizlioglu H, Baykan EC, Eryilmaz S, Inan B, Katircioglu SF, Ozyurda U. Effect of carbon dioxide insufflation on free internal thoracic artery flows: is it a vasodilator? *J Thorac Cardiovasc Surg.* 2004;128:354-6.

[181] Koramaz I, Ozkan M, Kesim M, Güven KY, Kadioglu M, Ulku C, Cobanoglu U, Yaris E, Kalyoncu NI, Ozcan F. The contracting and relaxing responses of human internal mammary artery grafts harvested by two different methods. *Pharmacol Res.* 2005;51:567-73.

[182] Tarhan A, Kehlibar T, Yapici F, Yilmaz M, Arslan Y, Yapici N, Ozler A. Role of physiological state 'normothermia' in internal thoracic artery spasm after harvesting. *Eur J Cardiothorac Surg.* 2006;30:749-52.

[183] Tarhan IA, Kehlibar T, Yilmaz M, Arslan Y, Dumantepe M, Berkoz K, Pancaroglu C, Ozler A. Normothermia is the key for the treatment of internal thoracic artery spasm. *Heart Surg Forum.* 2007;10:E180-5.

[184] Tarhan IA, Kehlibar T, Arslan Y, Yilmaz M, Dumantepe M, Berkoz K, Pancaroglu C, Ozler A. Effects of normothermic organ bath and verapamil-nitroglycerin solution alone or in combination on the blood flow of radial artery. *Eur J Cardiothorac Surg.* 2007;32:617-22.

[185] Mueed I, Tazzeo T, Doharris L, Aziz T, Chu V, Janssen LJ. Reduction of arterial graft smooth muscle mass by moderate heat therapy. *Transl Res.* 2011;157:128-38.

[186] Beşoğul Y. Endothoracic injection of room air for internal mammary artery harvest. *J Card Surg.* 2009n;24:309-11.

[187] Psacioğlu H, Atay Y, Cetindağ B, Saribülbül O, Buket S, Hamulu A. Easy harvesting of radial artery with ultrasonically activated scalpel. *Ann Thorac Surg.* 1998 ;65:984-5.].

[188] Ronan JW, Perry LA, Barner HB, Sundt TM 3rd. Radial artery harvest: comparison of ultrasonic dissection with standard technique. *Ann Thorac* Surg. 2000;69:113-4;

[189] Georghiou GP, Stamler A, Berman M, Sharoni E, Vidne BA, Sahar G. Advantages of the ultrasonic harmonic scalpel for radial artery harvesting. *Asian Cardiovasc Thorac Ann.* 2005;13:58-60;

[190] Canosa C, Nasso G, De Filippo CM, Modugno P, Spatuzza P, Calvo E, Testa N, Alessandrini F. Open clip-free radial artery harvesting with the harmonic shears. *J Card Surg.* 2007;22:139-41;

[191] Erkut B, Unlu Y, Karapolat S, Ugur Kocogullari C, Ceviz M, Becit N, Kocak H. Comparison of harmonic scalpel and high-frequency electrocautery in radial artery harvesting. *J Cardiovasc Surg (Torino).* 2008;49:371-9;

[192] Oz BS, Mataraci I, Iyem H, Kuralay E, Doganci S, Demirkilic U, Yokusoglu M, Tatar H. Comparison of ultrasonically activated scalpel and traditional technique in radial artery harvesting: clinical research. *Thorac Cardiovasc Surg.* 2007;55:104-7;

[193] Fawzy HF. Harvesting of the radial artery for coronary artery bypass grafting: comparison of ultrasonic harmonic scalpel dissector with the conventional technique. *J Card Surg.* 2009;24:285-9.

[194] Brazio PS, Laird PC, Xu C, Gu J, Burris NS, Brown EN, Kon ZN, Poston RS. Harmonic scalpel versus electrocautery for harvest of radial artery conduits: reduced risk of spasm and intimal injury on optical coherence tomography. *J Thorac Cardiovasc Surg.* 2008;136:1302-8.

[195] Brown EN, Burris NS, Kon ZN, Grant MC, Brazio PS, Xu C, Laird P, Gu J, Kallam S, Desai P, Poston RS. Intraoperative detection of intimal lipid in the radial artery predicts degree of postoperative spasm. *Atherosclerosis.* 2009;205:466-71.

[196] Burris NS, Brown EN, Grant M, Kon ZN, Gibber M, Gu J, Schwartz K, Kallam S, Joshi A, Vitali R, Poston RS. Optical coherence tomography imaging as a quality assurance tool for evaluating endoscopic harvest of the radial artery. *Ann Thorac Surg.* 2008;85:1271-7.

[197] Tector AJ, Schmahl TM, Crouch JD, Canino VR, Heckel RC. Sequential, free and Y internal thoracic artery grafts. *Eur Heart J.* 1989;10 Suppl H:71-7.

[198] Yildirim V, Akay HT, Bingol H, Bolcal C, Iyem H, Doğanci S, Demirkilic U, Tatar H. Pre-emptive stellate ganglion block increases the patency of radial artery grafts in coronary artery bypass surgery. *Acta Anaesthesiol Scand.* 2007;51:434-40.

[199] Kulshrestha P, Rao L, Garb JL, Rousou JA, Engelman RM, Wait RB. Use of extrafascially harvested radial artery for coronary artery revascularization: technical considerations. *J Card Surg.* 1999;14:26-31.

[200] Gaudiani VA, Buch WS, Chin AK, Ayres LJ, Fogarty TJ. An improved technique for the internal mammary artery coronary bypass graft procedure. *J Card Surg*. 1988;3:467-73.
[201] He GW, Taggart DP. Spasm in arterial grafts in coronary artery bypass grafting surgery. *Ann Thorac Surg*. 2016;101(3):1222-9. Epub 2015 Nov 14.
[202] He GW, Taggart DP. Antispastic management in arterial grafts in coronary artery bypass grafting surgery. *Ann Thorac Surg*. 2016 (in press).

In: Coronary Artery Disease
Editor: Courtney Burke

ISBN: 978-1-63485-330-9

Chapter 2

PERCUTANEOUS VERSUS SURGICAL CORONARY REVASCULARIZATION IN THE CURRENT ERA AND BEYOND: IS THE DEBATE OVER?

Sameer A. Hirji*, MD, Faith C. Robertson[2], BS, Kevin L. Anderson Jr[3], BS, and Ralf E. Harskamp[4], MD

[1]Department of Surgery, Brigham and Women's Hospital, Harvard Medical School, Boston, MA, US
[2]Harvard Medical School, Boston, MA, US
[3]Duke University School of Medicine, Durham, NC, US
[4]Academic Medical Center – University of Amsterdam, Amsterdam, the Netherlands

ABSTRACT

Coronary artery disease is a leading cause of morbidity and mortality in developed countries around the globe. Coronary revascularization, either with coronary artery bypass grafting (CABG) or percutaneous coronary intervention (PCI) has been shown to be safe and effective in appropriately selected patients. Both revascularization strategies have

* Corresponding author: Sameer A. Hirji, MD Address: Department of Surgery, Brigham and Women's Hospital, Harvard Medical chool, 75 Francis Street, Boston, MA 02115, US. Email: shirji@partners.org.

undergone significant advancements, creating the need to (re) examine data from clinical studies and critically scrutinize existing guidelines in order to determine the optimal care for each individual patient. In this chapter, we will discuss the CABG and PCI in the current era, and highlight relative strengths and weaknesses of each approach. We will also discuss various risk-stratification scoring systems, and consider both procedures in the context of different demographic populations, including advanced age, gender, acute coronary syndromes, previous CABG, renal failure, diabetes mellitus and left main involvement. The continued development of objective patient-assessment tools to offer patient-tailored recommendation is critical. Moreover, novel therapeutic approaches and treatment regimens, such as a hybrid strategy, as well as techniques targeted at improving stent and graft patency will be evaluated. This synthesis of information will provide an essential framework for evidence-based approach of coronary revascularization in the current era and beyond.

Keywords: PCI, CABG

Introduction

The pathophysiology of coronary artery disease (CAD) was first described in 1876, when Adam Hammer hypothesized that angina was caused by interruption of coronary blood supply and that myocardial infarction occurred after the occlusion of at least one coronary artery [1]. The concept of coronary revascularization is based on restoring blood flow either through bypassing the occluded sections or territories of coronary arteries using a conduit (vein or arterial graft) or through a catheter-based intraluminal expansion with balloon angioplasty with or without coronary stenting. This fundamental concept has persisted through decades and has widely become the standard of care for many patients with high-risk CAD and symptomatic CAD refractory to optimal medical therapy [2, 3].

Revascularization strategies, both coronary artery bypass graft (CABG) and percutaneous coronary intervention (PCI), are effective treatments for CAD in carefully selected patients, and are the most commonly performed operative procedures in cardiovascular care [4]. Based on recent data from the Center for Disease Control and Prevention (CDC), there were approximately 150,000 CABG procedures and 450,000 PCI procedures performed in the United States in 2012 [5].

Despite significant technical and technological advancements that have been made in both fields, there still exists a lack of consensus on identifying the superior approach on a patient-specific basis. Treatment decisions in the context of coronary disease vary according to the patient's preference, disease etiology, demographics and past medical history. In most cases, the decision-making process is complex, and can be particularly challenging in patients who are at increased risk for complications, including the elderly, those with diabetes, end stage renal disease, and complex multivessel CAD, specifically those with left main or multivessel disease involving the proximal left anterior descending (LAD) coronary artery. Thus, having a multi-disciplinary 'heart team' is absolutely essential to ensure treatment decisions are tailored to individual patient profile, cardiac function and extent of vessel disease.

With the advent of a variety of objective assessment tools and emergence of recent clinical trials, which will be addressed later in the chapter, treatment regimens are evolving and in some cases, becoming more specialized and patient-goal oriented, with the goal of optimizing outcomes and reducing costs. Recent evidence from clinical trials has also challenged some of the existing practice guidelines. This chapter will synthesize contemporary studies and practices to provide an essential framework for evidence-based approach of coronary revascularization in the current era and beyond.

Surgical Revascularization

The 1960s brought great advances in the treatment of CAD, beginning with Goetz and his colleagues in 1961, who are credited for performing the first successful human coronary artery bypass operation [6]. In 1964, Kolesov and his team performed the first successful internal mammary artery-coronary artery anastomosis, and Favoloro et al. reported using saphenous vein to restore coronary artery blood flow in 171 patients [1, 7, 8].

Through the years, numerous advancements and distinct approaches to reestablish perfusion to the myocardium have reduced morbidity, mortality, and need for extensive or additional revascularization [3, 9-11]. These include off-pump CABG, smaller incisions, enhanced myocardial preservation, and use of durable arterial conduits.

On-/Off-Pump CABG

Historically, most CABG procedures have been performed while on cardiopulmonary bypass. It was not until the late 1990s when interest in off-pump coronary artery bypass (OPCAB) surgery emerged and subsequently peaked. Initial results of OPCAB were promising with comparable results to on-pump CABG, as demonstrated in several large single center cohort studies [12, 13]. Reported benefits of OPCAB include lower rates of renal failure, cerebrovascular accidents (CVA), fewer cognitive deficits, less psychomotor defects, lower transfusion rates, and reduced systemic inflammation [14]. Subsequent randomized studies showed mixed results. In a recent meta-analytic study in which 59 randomized studies were included (n = 8,961), the authors found a 30% reduction in the occurrence of post-operative stroke in the group who underwent OPCAB; with similar outcomes for mortality or myocardial infarction [15]. OPCAB is still widely used today, particularly at some centers without the infrastructure for cardiopulmonary bypass.

Minimally Invasive CABG

More recent developments, such as minimally invasive, thoracoscopic and robotic assisted approaches have also influenced a surgeons approach to CAD treatment. These surgeries do not require cardiopulmonary bypass and are performed through smaller incisions. Benefits include reduced operative time, reduced recovery time, decreased need for blood transfusion, less time under anesthesia, and decreased length of ICU stay [16, 17]. The flipside of using these sternal-sparing operative techniques is a more limited operating field. As such, the indication for using these techniques is most often for bypassing isolated proximal LAD lesions, with the left internal mammary artery (LIMA) as the conduit of preference [1, 16, 18].

Arterial and Venous Conduits

In 2011, American Heart Association (AHA) Guidelines for Coronary Artery Bypass Graft Surgery advocated the use of arterial grafts for anastomosis to the LAD [19, 20]. The IMA grafts, in particular, are most preferred since they have consistently demonstrated long-term benefits, including lower failure rates in terms of patency over vein grafts in a diverse cohort of patients [21-23]. The reasons for IMA's superior patency and resiliency to atherosclerosis may be attributed to its relatively similar diameter to that of the LAD, which tends to limit flow turbulences that create frictional force and shear stress-induced endothelial injury, and the fact that the IMA graft has a protective muscular wall, which helps to reduce surgical trauma during harvesting, and a sufficient blood supply that helps to preserve the wall function [24]. The IMA can be harvested as a single (Left IMA or Right IMA) or bilateral graft (BIMA), and either as a pedicle or as a skeletonized graft. Of the various techniques, the skeletonized approach is postulated to reduce sternal devascularization and thereby minimize the risk of sternal infections, as well as improve overall conduit length [25, 26]. Importantly, however, the decision to use an IMA should be carefully considered taking into account the extent of stenosis of the target vessel. For instance, in a recent analysis of the frequency and predictors of internal mammary graft failure from the PREVENT IV (Project of Ex-vivo Vein graft Engineering via Transfection IV) trial by Harskamp et al., IMA failure was associated with higher rates of repeat revascularization, and more likely to occur in patients with intermediate LAD stenosis (<75%), or those that underwent additional bypass grafting to the diagonal branches [27].

In recent years, there is emerging evidence to demonstrate the superior efficacy and safety of BIMA, with a reported survival advantage as high as 15% at 15 years [28, 29]. While the procedure can be technically challenging and perhaps time consuming depending on the surgeon's experience, BIMA grafting has been shown to be favorable in women, elderly, diabetics, and select patients with left ventricular and renal disease [28, 30-32].

In addition to the IMA, other arteries and veins can be used as conduits. Reversed saphenous vein grafts (SVGs) are most commonly used for bypassing non-LAD lesions. However, a major disadvantage is their declining patency with time, with studies suggesting graft failure rates of >50% after 10 years [33, 34]. There are 3 major mechanisms than can cause vein graft failure: acute thrombosis, neo-intimal hyperplasia, and accelerated atherosclerosis. Some proposed preventative mechanisms to mitigate this issue of graft failure include matching and quality assessment of conduit and target vessel, lipid-lowering drugs, antithrombotic therapy, and cessation of smoking [33, 34]. The utility of radial artery grafts is much debated partly because they are very prone to spasm [35]. In some instances, the gastro-epiploic artery has also been used particularly to bypass the lesions in the right coronary artery or its branches, although it is also prone to spasm [36].

PERCUTANEOUS REVASCULARIZATION

The origins of percutaneous coronary intervention (PCI) can be traced to 1964, when Charles Dotter and Melvin Judkins had suggested and successfully demonstrated the use of prosthetic device (specifically guide wire and coaxial Teflon catheters) inside the peripheral arteries of the leg to maintain blood flow following dilation [37]. The first successful coronary balloon angioplasty was performed in 1977 on an awake human in Zurich, Switzerland by Andreas Grüntzig [38]. Grüntzig expanded a non-branching section of the LAD, with an eighty percent stenosis. On the 10-year anniversary of this procedure, the patient's LAD narrowing was reexamined and the vessel remained almost perfectly expanded. After his initial efforts in 1977, Grüntzig presented his next four angioplasty cases at the American Heart Association, earning peer recognition for his pioneering work [38]. These initial efforts spurred genuine interest among various clinicians and investors to transform the field of percutaneous revascularization, beginning with advent of balloon-expandable stents in the 1980s [38].

Numerous studies and clinical trials throughout the 1990s showed the superiority of stent placement over balloon angioplasty. Notably, it reduced rates of restenosis, acute coronary artery closure, and emergency CABG. By the late 1990s, stents, particularly bare metal (BMS) ones, were used in almost 84% of percutaneous coronary interventions (i.e., those done via a catheter, and not by open-chest surgery) [10, 38, 39]. The main concern of coronary stents, however, was centered on the risk of early thrombosis, which resulted in stent occlusion. To remedy this issue, improvements in stent designs ensued to ensure full apposition to the arterial wall. These inventions were further combined with significant advancements in drug therapy, involving the routine use of aspirin, with platelet aggregation inhibitors such as clopidogrel, ticagrelor, and presugrel [38].

In recent years, the advent of drug-eluting stents has helped to reduce the relatively high rate of restenosis and subsequent need for repeat revascularizations that was observed with BMS. As high as 50% to 70% reduction in target lesion revascularization by DES compared to BMS has been demonstrated consistently in multiple clinical trials, including the SIRIUS, RAVEL, SCANDSTENT, TAXUS IV, and TAXUS V trials [40-43]. Most of these studies however, have looked at first generation DES stents, which are either sirolimus-eluting (SES) or paclitaxel-eluting (PES). Only a few have looked at 2nd generation everolimus-eluting (EES) or zotarolimus-eluting stents (ZES), namely the SPIRIT FIRST (1) trial, and ENDEAVOR group of trials, respectively [44].

While restenosis of stents usually occurs within the first year after stent placement, where DES are superior to BMS, late restenosis (after 1 year) has been observed in all types of stents, with reported rates of 1 to 2% [45-47]. Patients who prematurely discontinue dual antiplatelet therapy are more vulnerable to stent thrombosis and the resultant high associated mortality, which is reportedly between 20% and 45% [48, 49]. Current consensus in clinical practice is to treat these DES patients with at least 12 months of dual antiplatelet therapy to avoid late stent thrombosis [48]. Compliance to drug therapies following stent placement is absolutely critical and must be carefully assessed in patients prior to the procedure. Current guidelines emphasize this concern and recommend discussion prior to implantation of DES, regarding the need for and duration of dual antiplatelet therapy, and ability of patient to comply with and tolerate the therapy for the duration indicated *(Class I; Level of Evidence: C)* [19, 50].

RISK STRATIFICATION OF PATIENTS WITH CAD

Risk stratification of patients in the setting of CAD is currently evidence based, with clinical risk - in terms of mortality and other risk factors- assessed using the Society of Thoracic Surgeons (STS) score or the European System for Cardiac operative Risk Evaluation (EuroSCORE), and angiographic risk-based solely on anatomical features- assessed using the SYNergy between PCI with TAXUS and Cardiac Surgery Score (SYNTAX) data [51]. These scoring systems, particularly the SYNTAX score, have greatly improved patient selection and optimized revascularization strategies for high-risk patients [51]. Briefly, the Synergy between PCI with Taxus and Cardiac Surgery (SYNTAX) trial was intended to formulate a model to facilitate objective decision making regarding an optimal CAD treatment strategy [52, 53]. SYNTAX was a prospective randomized control study that encompassed 85 different medical centers, and was very unique in that it had an "all-comers" design involving the consecutive enrollment of all eligible patients with three-vessel or left main coronary artery disease [2]. While patient outcomes coincided with previous studies- in that CABG offered a survival advantage along with a decreased requirement for a repeat intervention up to 4 years after revascularization - these results allowed generation of an angiographic tool for grading the complexity of CAD and guidelines for treatment [53-55]. Overall, the SYNTAX score has acceptable reproducibility on the one-year outcome of those having PCI, but lacks the ability to determine the effect on the same outcome following surgical revascularization [10, 54]. To widen the application of the SYNTAX score and improve its diagnostic accuracy, the SYNTAX Score II was eventually designed and subsequently validated to ensure its robustness. The SYNTAX Score II combines the anatomical based SYNTAX score with clinical variables, including presence of unprotected LM disease, female gender, chronic obstructive pulmonary disease, age, and left ventricular ejection fraction. This updated version allows for improved decision-making, to a greater degree, between CABG and PCI [56-59].

The EuroSCORE, on the other hand, was published in 1999 and assesses 17-risk factors, which include a combination of patient-related, cardiac related and surgery related variables, previously developed from a large European data set [60, 61]. The latest edition of the EUROSCORE II, validated in 2011, has better operative mortality discrimination compared to the original EuroSCORE, which reportedly overestimated the predicted risk of operative mortality. This newer version, takes into account additional clinically relevant risk variables such as New York Heart Association (NYHA) status, elective, urgent, emergency, or salvage surgery, preoperative dialysis and insulin-dependent diabetes [62].

Likewise, the STS score was published in 2007 and predicts postoperative mortality, and other outcomes (length of stay, sternal wound infection, renal failure, and so on) in patients undergoing open-heart surgery [63]. While both models have good calibration and discrimination, recent studies have shown that the EuroSCORE II is more inclusive and has more flexibility when dealing with patients undergoing very complex procedures. Thus, for many clinicians, the EuroSCORE is often considered the gold standard model against which other recent models are validated [51, 62, 64].

Accurate prediction of patient risks for various cardiac procedures is essential and increasingly important today from a surgical and hospital outcomes standpoint. In most cases, a combination of score components from the EuroSCORE, STS as well as SYNTAX is used to identify high-risk patients and appropriately select interventional strategies with either PCI or CABG, or both.

COMPARING SURGICAL VERSUS PERCUTANEOUS REVASCULARIZATION

Treatment decisions in the context of coronary artery disease are often complex, and involve a comprehensive assessment of disease etiology, patient risk factors including age, diabetes, end stage renal disease, and complex CAD (single versus multivessel), as well as procedure related challenges. In a majority of patients either CABG or PCI is a clear choice – and is reflected in existing guidelines- but in some instances, there is equipoise. In these circumstances, a multi-disciplinary 'heart team' helps facilitate evidence-based treatment decisions, which are tailored to individual patient profile, cardiac function and extent of vessel disease. The heart team, which is comprised of interventional cardiologist and a cardiac surgeon, is responsible for objectively reviewing the patient's medical condition and coronary anatomy, and determining whether that PCI and/or CABG are technically feasible and reasonable.

Patients with Left Anterior Descending Artery Disease

For the management of LAD disease, current AHA guidelines recommend CABG with a left internal mammary artery (LIMA) graft to improve survival, particularly in patients with significant (≥70% diameter) stenosis in the proximal LAD artery and evidence of extensive ischemia (*Class IIa; Level of Evidence: B*) [50]. These guidelines were based on a number of cohort studies in the 1990s. For instance, an early landmark study by Loop et al. examining outcomes of IMA grafting alone or combined with one or more saphenous vein grafts for LAD disease in 2306 patients found a 93.4% 10-year survival rate compared to 88% in patients who had received only the saphenous vein graft [65]. Likewise, another more recent study by Smith et al. examining over 18000 patients with significant (>75% stenosis) CAD found a superior survival advantage for CABG over PCI or medical management alone [66]. Recent cohort studies and RCTs, however, showed that PCI and CABG result in similar survival rates in this patient population [50, 67, 68]. In a recent meta-analysis of two RCTs and two observational studies looking at outcomes of CABG versus PCI in proximal LAD disease by Harskamp et al., the incidence of cardiac mortality and MI was similar between the groups although patients who underwent a CABG had lower target vessel revascularization [69]. Existing guidelines state that either a CABG or PCI to improve survival is beneficial in survivors of sudden cardiac death with presumed ischemia-mediated ventricular tachycardia caused by significant (≥70% diameter) stenosis in a major coronary artery (*Class IIA; CABG Level of Evidence: B; PCI Level of Evidence: C*) [50].

Patients with Right Coronary or Circumflex Disease

For isolated single vessel disease in these territories, PCI is often preferred to CABG, as it helps to reduce the morbidity associated with the CABG procedure. However, there is also little data available as well as absence of definitive evidence to suggest outcomes are better with CABG for these lesions. Current recommendations suggest that CABG or PCI to improve symptoms is beneficial in patients with 1 or more significant (≥70% diameter) coronary artery stenoses amenable to revascularization and unacceptable angina despite medical treatment (*Class I; Level of Evidence: A*) [50]. Patients in whom CABG is reasonable include those with a large amount of ischemic myocardium, those with right dominant coronary supply, those who are not candidates for long-term dual antiplatelet therapy, and finally those that have failed prior PCI [20, 50].

Patients with Left Main Artery Disease

Current AHA guidelines on the management of LM disease mostly favor CABG. Specifically, CABG to improve survival is recommended for patients with significant (>50% diameter stenosis) LM stenosis. On the other hand, PCI is appropriate and reasonable for unprotected LM disease in a patient with unstable angina or NSTEMI who is not a candidate for CABG *(Class I; Level of Evidence: B)* [19, 50]. These guidelines are based on various landmark studies, a few of them outlined in Table 1 below. Importantly, however, recently published studies have challenged some of these guidelines and demonstrated similar clinical outcomes following revascularization, although stenting has been associated with significantly higher need for target-vessel revascularization compared to CABG [70, 71]. In a recent large published RCT (n = 600 patients) by Ahn et al., the Premier of Randomized Comparison of Bypass Surgery vs. Angioplasty Using Sirolimus-Eluting Stent in patients with Left Main Coronary Artery Disease (PRECOMBAT) study, there was no difference in the rate of MACCE events between these patient groups at 5 year follow-up [72]. Furthermore, data from a recent meta-analysis that compared randomized clinical trials indicate that PCI with DES stenting yields similar outcomes 1-year and 2-year follow- up in terms of major adverse cardiac events (MACE) in selected, low risk patients with left main coronary artery disease [73].

Management of LM disease can be challenging at times and with recent evidence showing the feasibility of PCI in carefully selected patients. Current AHA guidelines also advocate for a heart Team approach to revascularization in patients with unprotected left main or complex CAD (*Class I, Level of Evidence: C*) [50, 74]. Because lesion location is an important determinant when considering PCI or CABG for unprotected LM CAD, existing guidelines also advocate for calculation of the Society of Thoracic Surgeons (STS) and SYNTAX scores to assess patients with unprotected left main and complex CAD (*Class IIa; Level of Evidence:* B) [50, 74].

Table 1. Summary of outcomes of recent Randomized clinical trials comparing PCI and CABG for the treatment of Left Main Coronary Artery Disease

STUDY	No of Patients	Follow-up, Time, Y	Primary Endpoint	PCI	CABG	P-value
Buszman et al. 2009 (LE MANS) [75]	53	1	Death, MI, Stroke, TVR	3.30%	0.50%	0.05
Park et al. 2011 (PRECOMBAT) [76]	600	1	Death, MI, Stroke, TVR	8.70%	6.70%	0.01 (non-inferiority)
Boudriot et al. 2011 [77]	201	1	Death, MI, TVR	19.00%	13.90%	0.19 (non-inferiority)
Morice et al. 2010 (SYNTAX) [78]	701	1	Death, MI, Stroke, TVR	15.80%	14%	0.440
Mohr et al. 2013 (SYNTAX) [79]	701	5	Death, MI, Stroke, TVR	46.50%	46.50%	0.010
Ahn et al. 2015 (PRECOMBAT) [72]	600	5	Death, MI, Stroke, TVR	17.50%	14.30%	0.260
Buszman et al. 2016 (LE MANS) [80]	105	10	Death, MI, Stroke, TVR	51.10%	64.40%	0.280

CABG- coronary artery bypass grafting, PCI – percutaneous coronary intervention, MI – myocardial infarction, TVR – target vessel revascularization.

Patients with Multivessel Disease

Multivessel coronary artery disease (MVD) is defined by significant atherosclerosis (>70% occlusion) involving at least two or three of the epicardial coronary arteries, and it occurs in 40-65% of patients with acute myocardial infarction [81]. MVD is associated with a higher burden of comorbidities and left ventricular dysfunction, and it significantly increases the risk of morbidity and mortality after interventional therapy [81-83]. Numerous studies on MVD have compared CABG to the various methods of PCI, from balloon angioplasty and bare metal stents, to first- and second-generation drug-eluting stents, and conclusions have fluctuated with time.

Current guidelines recommend either CABG or PCI to improve symptoms in patients with 1 or more significant (≥70% diameter) coronary artery stenoses amenable to revascularization (*Class 1A; Level of Evidence: A*), and in patients with complex 3-vessel CAD (e.g., SYNTAX score >22), with or without involvement of the proximal LAD artery who are good candidates for CABG (*Class IIA; Level of Evidence: B*). However, these guidelines recommend CABG in patients with significant (≥70% diameter) stenoses in 3 major coronary arteries (with or without involvement of the proximal LAD artery) or in the proximal LAD plus 1 other major coronary artery (*Class I, Level of Evidence: B*) [19, 50]. These guidelines were based on conclusions drawn from multiple RCTs and large clinical registries to ensure enough statistical power and confidence (Table 2).

Other important clinical trials investigating outcomes of PCI versus CABG in multivessel CAD are worth mentioning. These include the Arterial Revascularization Therapies Study Part I [ARTS I], the Medicine, Angioplasty, or Surgery Study for Multivessel Coronary Artery Disease [MASS II], and the Argentine Randomized Study of Coronary Angioplasty with Stenting versus Coronary Bypass Surgery in Patients with Multiple Vessel Disease [ERACI-II] [84]. In these studies, which specifically compared bare metal stenting PCI to CABG, negligible difference was noted in long-term survival rates [1, 10, 85]. However, secondary outcomes from these trials revealed an increased need for revascularization after 5 years with bare metal stenting, or in other words, less frequent need with CABG [84, 85]. With the advent of DES, findings of some of these trials (e.g., ARTS I) are not relevant to current practice today because DES, in comparison to BMS, have been shown to reduce the rate of both angiographic restenosis and repeat revascularization, a previously well known limitation of PCI [40].

Table 2. Summary of Outcomes of Important Randomized Clinical Trials and large observational studies comparing PCI and CABG for the treatment of Multivessel CAD

STUDY	No of Patients	Follow-up, Time, Y	Primary Endpoint	PCI	CABG	P-value
BARI Investigators. 2007 (BARI) [92]	1827	10	Mortality	29.00%	26.50%	0.18
Booth et al. 2008 (SoS) [87]	988	6	Mortality	10.90%	6.80%	0.02
Hueb et al. 2010 (MASS II) [93]	611	10	Mortality	23.90%	25.10%	0.09
Serruys et al. 2009 (SYNTAX) [2]	1800	1	Mortality	4.40%	3.50%	0.37
Mohr et al. 2013 (SYNTAX) [79]	1800	5	Mortality	13.90%	11.40%	0.10
Park et al. 2015 (BEST) [94]	880	2	Death, MI, TVR	11.00%	7.90%	0.32 (non-inferiority)
Park et al. 2015 (BEST) [94]	880	4.6	Death, MI, TVR	15.30%	10.60%	0.04
Bangalore S et al. 2015 [95]	18446	2.9	Mortality	3.10%	2.90%	0.50
Bangalore S et al. 2015 (with CKD) [96]	11305	4	Mortality	22.70%	20.50%	0.04

CABG- coronary artery bypass grafting, PCI – percutaneous coronary intervention, MI – myocardial infarction, TVR – target vessel revascularization.

There are also several trials comparing drug eluting stent PCI (with DES) and CABG that are noteworthy. A few of these include the FREEDOM trial, SYNTAX trial, VA CARDS, and CARDia (Table 3) [84]. These studies have consistently demonstrated a higher rate of stroke but a lower mortality rate with CABG, and a higher rate of repeat revascularization with PCI [2, 86]. Furthermore, comparing first generation drug-eluting stents to CABG in the Stent on Surgery (SOS) trial, Booth and colleagues showed a continuing survival advantage after 6 years for patients who had a CABG [87]. PCI consistently reduced hospital mortality in all age groups [88]. CABG patients experienced greater relief from angina than those undergoing PCI, though the difference was minimal [89]. The ASCERT (American College of Cardiology Foundation and the Society of Thoracic Surgeons Collaboration on the Comparative Effectiveness of Revascularization Strategies) published in the New England Journal of Medicine showed that even though CABG had better outcomes over a period of four years (16.4% versus 20.8%; risk ratio 0.779), it did so with a higher financial burden than PCI [90]. In 2015, an observational registry study in New York compared second-generation DES to CABG ($n = 9223$ matched pairs). This study found that PCI with evorlimus-eluding stents had a lower risk of death and stroke within 30 days of the procedure, though there was no difference long-term (>30 days). PCI was also associated with greater risk of myocardial infarction in patients with incomplete revascularization, and a need for future revascularization [91].

Patients with Acute Coronary Syndrome (ACS)

In patients presenting with ACS, PCI is generally the preferred initial treatment surgery for the culprit lesion in STEMI with a goal of timely restoration of blood flow to the occluded territories in the coronary tree. Current guidelines recommend primary PCI within 12 hours of onset of STEMI *(Class I; Level of Evidence: A)* and should be performed within 90 minutes of presenting to a hospital with PCI capabilities *(Class I; Level of Evidence: B)* [19, 50, 97]. In the setting of NSTEMI or unstable angina, the impetus for revascularization is stronger to reduce symptoms and because myocardial ischemia occurring in the context of ACS is critical and potentially life threatening. In a multicenter British randomized clinical trial (RITA 3) comparing interventional versus conservative treatments in 1800 patients with UA/NSTEMI, refractory or severe angina symptoms were notably halved with the interventional strategy, with no increased risk of death of MI [98]. In the setting of ACS and UA/NSTEMI, therefore, either CABG or PCI procedures are complementary and often utilized on case-by-case basis, taking into account the acuity of clinical presentation, extent of ischemia, and feasibility to achieve adequate or complete revascularization [98]. This is reflected in the current guidelines, which recommend an early invasive strategy with intent to perform revascularization in UA/NSTEMI patients who have refractory angina or hemodynamic or electrical instability, without contraindications *(Class I; Level of Evidence: B)* [19, 50].

Moreover, in the recent ACUITY (Acute Catheterization and Urgent Intervention Triage Strategy) trial by Ben-Gal and his colleagues, which compared outcomes of surgical versus percutaneous revascularization for multivessel disease in patients with ACS, PCI rather then CABG had lower rates of peri-procedural stroke, MI, major bleeding, and renal injury with comparable 1-month and 1 year rates of mortality. However, PCI was associated with an increased frequency of recurrent ischemia requiring additional repeat revascularization procedures at a later date [99]. In most cases, CABG is usually utilized in the setting of cardiogenic shock or PCI failure in the presence of ongoing ischemia, hemodynamic compromise, unfavorable anatomy, extensive multivessel disease, and in those patients that require concurrent repair of post-infarction mechanical complication of MI, such as ventricular septal rupture, or mitral valve insufficiency in the setting of papillary muscle rupture [19, 50].

Choice of Coronary Revascularization in Special Subgroups

Older Patients

The elderly patient population requires special attention, because of increased risk of mortality and perioperative complications (i.e., major bleeding and stroke) with revascularization in the setting of multiple comorbidities. Weintraub et al. investigated elderly patients and determined that after 4 years there was lower mortality as well as a long term survival advantage with CABG than with PCI in patients 65 years and older with two- or three-vessel coronary artery disease without acute myocardial infarction [100]. A 2009 meta-analysis of 10 clinical trials also reported lower mortality rated with CABG intervention than PCI for those greater than 65 years [101]. In a population of octogenarians, Singh et al. determined that the mortality rate was five times higher in comparison to the younger population and actually represents thirty percent of all deaths after PCI [88]. The author goes on to comment that in other studies age was actually an independent predictor of outcomes after percutaneous revascularization overall [88].

Gender

While the majority of patients with coronary artery disease are men, CAD is also the leading cause of death in women [88, 102, 103], yet women receive less revascularization and evidence-based medications [102]. In a population-based cohort study that spanned a decade, Guru et al. showed that women have a more complex clinical preoperative presentation and unfortunately are more likely to be readmitted with unstable angina and congestive heart failure after CABG, despite having similar survival rates compared to men [103]. Some studies, such as the one by Lempereur et al., that examined the risk factors for in-hospital mortality following PCI, female sex remained an independent predictor of mortality [104]. Furthermore, in evaluating DES versus BMS angioplasty, while there is a profound prognostic advantage for both genders, female patients reportedly had a higher benefit [105].

Previous CABG

In patients that have previously undergone a CABG procedure, additional PCI procedures for isolated disease is feasible but can be sometimes challenging. Current AHA guidelines state that PCI is reasonable in patients with previous CABG, 1 or more significant (≥70% diameter) coronary artery stenoses associated with ischemia, and unacceptable angina despite medical management (*Class IIa; Level of Evidence: C*). However, these guidelines further state that the usefulness of CABG or PCI to improve survival is uncertain in patients with previous CABG and extensive anterior wall ischemia on noninvasive testing (*Class IIb; Level of Evidence: B*) [19, 50]. Several cohort studies examining revascularization procedures following initial CABG have shown similar rates of mid- and long-term survival 2 years after the procedure. In certain patients however, such as those with multi-vessel disease unsuitable for PCI, multiple number of diseased grafts, availability of patent IMA conduits and good distal targets for bypass placements, the choice of repeat CABG can be justified. According to one study by Brener et al., which examined predictors of revascularization method (either CABG or PCI) in patients with previous CABG, the choice of CABG was driven more by anatomical rather than clinical characteristics, and the most important predictors for mortality were higher age and lower ejection fraction [106]. PCI, on the other hand, is often utilized in patients with suitable PCI targets, a patent graft to the LAD artery or in those with extensive comorbidities, which make them high-risk candidates for CABG [106]. Weintraub et al. showed that even though the initial mortality was higher for CABG, there was little difference long term, and more patients required additional procedures following a PCI [107]. Likewise, Stephan et al. retrospectively analyzed 632 patients with previous CABG, and found that complete revascularization was achieved in 38% of patients who underwent PCI versus 92% in those that underwent re-CABG [108]. In fact, the study further demonstrated that either procedure had equivalent overall survival, and event free survival at 6 years follow up, although PCI was associated with lower procedural morbidity [108]. A more recent study, a five-year non-randomized retrospective study of patients who experienced graft failure, echoed these findings and demonstrated repeat revascularization occurred more frequently after BMS PCI implantation than any other process [109].

Renal Failure

Kidney function is an important clinical parameter to assess when considering coronary revascularization. Chronic renal disease and renal failure are common sequalae of CAD and increase patients' risk of procedure-related morbidity and mortality [110, 111]. Additionally, patients with end stage renal disease have a much greater incidence of CAD and acute myocardial infarction [112, 113]. Hemmelgarn et al. evaluated survival in patients who received CABG, PCI or no revascularization for three stratifications of kidney function: dialysis-dependent kidney disease, non-dialysis-dependent kidney disease, and a group with serum creatinine above 2.3 mg/dL (reference group) [114]. Based on their data, CABG was associated with increased survival in all groups of kidney disease, while PCI was superior to the no-revascularization group particularly in the reference group patients and the dialysis-dependent group [114]. This study was further validated by Krishnaswami et al. in which CABG is more favorable than PCI with stenting, primarily due to a low re-operation rate, despite a higher level of invasiveness and longer recovery time [115]. Despite these results however, a recent assessment of nationwide trends in revascularization for patients with end stage renal disease showed that PCI intervention for a ST-elevation myocardial infarction has increased from 18.6% to 37.8% between 2003 and 2011; CABG had decreased slightly, 6.1% to 5.7% [116]. Importantly, accurate dosing of antiplatelet and anti-thrombin drugs in patients with CKD should be ensured to avoid under-dosing, which could increase the likelihood of stent thrombosis and/or complications.

Diabetes Mellitus

Several trials have examined revascularization strategies in patients with diabetes mellitus (DM) and multivessel coronary disease (Table 3). The first large trial comparing CABG and PCI exclusively in diabetic patients was the FREEDOM trial, which showed superiority of CABG to PCI with drug eluting stents in terms of long-term mortality [117]. As many subsequent trials were too small to reach consensus, a recent meta-analysis by Verma et al. (2013) examined eight randomized control trials of patients with diabetes mellitus and multivessel vascular disease to compare outcomes undergoing CABG or PCI [84]. At five years follow-up, all cause mortality was nearly one-third less in patients undergoing CABG. There was no significant difference seen at 1-year, and no difference in incidence of non-fatal myocardial infarction between the two groups. However, the relative risk of stroke after CABG was 2.4 times that of PCI patients (PCI risk of 0.8%). While CABG currently appears to be a superior technique to PCI in the diabetic subgroup, the impact of covariates on this decision remains uncertain. Comparing patients with insulin-treated diabetes mellitus with non-insulin treated patients, a subgroup analysis of the FREEDOM trial study found minimal difference in PCI versus CABG [118]. Thus, factors such as insulin use, gender, age, and comorbidities should be taken into consideration when assessing treatment options for CAD in patients with diabetes.

Table 3. Summary of Outcomes of Recent Trials and large observational studies comparing PCI and CABG for the treatment of multivessel CAD in Diabetic patients

STUDY	No of Patients	Follow-up, Time, Y	Primary Endpoint	PCI	CABG	P-value
BARI investigators. 2007 (BARI) [92]	353	10	Mortality	54.50%	42.20%	0.03
Kapur et al. 2010 (CARDIa) [119]	502	1	Mortality	3.20%	3.20%	0.97
Farkouh et al. 2012 (FREEDOM) [120]	1900	5	Mortality	16.30%	10.90%	0.05
Kappetein et al. 2013 (SYNTAX) [121]	452	5	Mortality	19.50%	12.90%	0.07
Kamalesh et al. 2013 (Veterans Affairs Study) [122]	198	2	Mortality	21%	5%	N/A

Future Directions

Treatment patterns of coronary artery disease either through PCI or CABG have evolved significantly over the last decade, especially with the advent of more sophisticated stent technology, such bio-absorbable vascular scaffolds, novel antiplatelet agents, robust imaging and surgical platforms, as well as reliable extracorporeal circulatory support devices. Likewise, in recent years, institutional experiences have also grown resulting in better outcomes and improved efficacies of both these procedures. At the same time, there is also widespread interest among clinicians to minimize surgical trauma and improve techniques to further improve graft patency following CABG procedures. This has been achieved via standardization of routine surgical procedures, and use of buffered saline graft preservation solutions [123]. For instance, a recent study examining data from the Project of Ex-Vivo Vein Graft Engineering via Transfection IV (PREVENT IV) trial – a phase 3, multicenter, randomized, double-blind, placebo-controlled trial that enrolled 3014 patients at 107 US sites- vein grafts preserved in buffered saline solution had a lower vein graft failure rates and trended towards better long-term clinical outcomes compared with patients whose grafts were preserved in saline only or blood-based solutions [34].

The field of hybrid coronary revascularization (HCR)- involving simultaneous or staged PCI/CABG procedures in select patients- has also emerged in recent years with comparable and promising outcomes to CABG alone [124]. Typically, these procedures entail combining grafting the LAD with LIMA and stenting of non-LAD territory. In a recent survey among 200 cardiologists and cardiac surgeons from 100 top-ranked US hospitals, more than 75% of responders felt that HCR is a reasonable alternative technique for coronary revascularization among suitable patients (including older and relatively healthy patient population without complex lesions). Most predicted that the use of HCR would increase in the next decade [125]. In fact, current AHA guidelines state that HCR is reasonable in patients with limitations to traditional CABG (for instance, poor targets for CABG or calcified proximal aorta), those with lack of suitable graft conduits, and those with an unfavorable LAD artery for PCI due to either vessel tortuosity or chronic total occlusion *(Class IIa; Level of evidence: B)* [19, 50]. While the current state of HCR is still limited to selected patients, with increasing engagement from and dialogue between the interventionists and surgical communities, as well as validated data from RCTs, HCR has the possibility of becoming a reliable revascularization strategy in the upcoming years.

An important limitation of coronary angiography, which has been well described in previous studies, is that it tends to either under- or overestimate lesion stenosis [126]. In the last decade, physiological measurement techniques, such as an assessment of fractional flow reserve (FFR) or hyperemic trans-lesional pressure ratio, have been developed to improve the diagnostic accuracy and optimize treatment decisions. Historically, most studies have defined 'significant stenosis' as ≥70% diameter narrowing of a particular vessel. This is equivalent to an FFR ≤0.80, which is the ratio of maximal blood flow in a stenotic artery to normal maximal flow. A recent large randomized multicenter clinical trial, FAME [FFR versus Angiography for Multivessel Evaluation]) found that a physiologically guided approach was superior to the standard angiographically guided approach for percutaneous revascularization in patients with multivessel coronary artery disease [127]. Furthermore, the correlation of ischemia on stress testing with FFR values of <0.75 has been reported to have a high sensitivity (88%), specificity (100%), positive predictive value (100%), and overall accuracy (93%) [126]. In fact, current guidelines state that FFR is reasonable to assess angiographic intermediate coronary lesions (50% to 70% diameter stenosis) and can be useful for guiding revascularization decisions in symptomatic patients (*Class IIa; Level of Evidence: A*) [19, 50]. This is a new era in the percutaneous as well as surgical revascularization where increasingly more clinicians are utilizing a combination of angiographic as well as FFR based measurement techniques in their decision making process.

CONCLUSION

The recent decade has experienced significant advancements in the field coronary revascularization. With advancements in various assessment tools and in light of recent clinical trial results, current guidelines have been challenged in many ways, and ought to change to reflect current evidence and practices. There is also a myriad of treatment options available for coronary revascularization, highlighted above, together emphasizing the ever increased need for targeted patient selection, and further open dialogue between the various stakeholders involved in a multidisciplinary heart team. To some extent, technological advancements have improved the overall diagnostic accuracy, although there is lack of widespread utilization, partly due to lack of infrastructure, and lack of long-term evidence to justify these innovations. While this is a work in progress, further trials must be designed to focus on specific areas where optimal therapy has yet to be substantiated. Some of these include, FFR guided interventions, hybrid coronary revascularization, graft flow measurements, as well as minimally invasive CABG. This chapter highlights contemporary studies and practices, and helps to provide an essential framework for evidence-based approach of coronary revascularization in the current era and beyond.

REFERENCES

[1] Diodato, M. and Chedrawy, E.G., Coronary artery bypass graft surgery: the past, present, and future of myocardial revascularisation. *Surg Res Pract*, 2014. 2014: p. 726158.

[2] Serruys, P.W., Morice, M.C., Kappetein, A.P. et al., Percutaneous coronary intervention versus coronary-artery bypass grafting for severe coronary artery disease. *N Engl J Med*, 2009. 360(10): p. 961-972.

[3] Buxton, B.F., Komeda, M., Fuller, J.A. et al., Bilateral internal thoracic artery grafting may improve outcome of coronary artery surgery. Risk-adjusted survival. *Circulation*, 1998. 98(19 Suppl.): p. Ii1-6.

[4] Fingar, K.R., Stocks, C., Weiss, A.J. et al., Most Frequent Operating Room Procedures Performed in US Hospitals, 2003-2012: *Statistical Brief #186, in Healthcare Cost and Utilization Project (HCUP) Statistical Briefs*. 2014, Agency for Health Care Policy and Research (US): Rockville (MD).

[5] National Center for Health Statistics. Health, United States, 2014: With Special Feature on Adults Aged 55-64. Hyattsville, MD. 2015.

[6] Goetz, R.H., Rohman, M., Haller, J.D. et al., Internal mammary-coronary artery anastomosis. A nonsuture method employing tantalum rings. *J Thorac Cardiovasc Surg*, 1961. 41: p. 378-386.

[7] Proudfit, W.L., Shirey, E.K., and Sones, F.M., Jr., Selective cine coronary arteriography. Correlation with clinical findings in 1,000 patients. *Circulation*, 1966. 33(6): p. 901-910.

[8] Olearchyk, A.S., Vasilii I. Kolesov. A pioneer of coronary revascularization by internal mammary-coronary artery grafting. *J Thorac Cardiovasc Surg*, 1988. 96(1): p. 13-18.

[9] Flynn, M., Reddy, S., Shepherd, W. et al., Fast-tracking revisited: routine cardiac surgical patients need minimal intensive care. *Eur J Cardiothorac Surg*, 2004. 25(1): p. 116-122.

[10] Serruys, P.W., Kutryk, M.J., and Ong, A.T., Coronary-artery stents. *N Engl J Med,* 2006. 354(5): p. 483-495.

[11] Janssen, D.P., Noyez, L., Wouters, C. et al., Preoperative prediction of prolonged stay in the intensive care unit for coronary bypass surgery. *Eur J Cardiothorac Surg*, 2004. 25(2): p. 203-207.

[12] Benetti, F.J., Naselli, G., Wood, M. et al., Direct myocardial revascularization without extracorporeal circulation. Experience in 700 patients. *Chest*, 1991. 100(2): p. 312-316.

[13] Buffolo, E., de Andrade, C.S., Branco, J.N. et al., Coronary artery bypass grafting without cardiopulmonary bypass. *Ann Thorac Surg*, 1996. 61(1): p. 63-66.

[14] Moller, C.H., Penninga, L., Wetterslev, J. et al., Off-pump versus on-pump coronary artery bypass grafting for ischaemic heart disease. *Cochrane Database Syst Rev*, 2012. 3: p. Cd007224.

[15] Afilalo, J., Rasti, M., Ohayon, S.M. et al., Off-pump vs. on-pump coronary artery bypass surgery: an updated meta-analysis and meta-regression of randomized trials. *Eur Heart J*, 2012. 33(10): p. 1257-1267.

[16] Deppe, A.C., Liakopoulos, O.J., Kuhn, E.W. et al., Minimally invasive direct coronary bypass grafting versus percutaneous coronary intervention for single-vessel disease: a meta-analysis of 2885 patients. *Eur J Cardiothorac Surg*, 2015. 47(3): p. 397-406; discussion 406.

[17] Benedetto, U., Raja, S.G., Soliman, R.F. et al., Minimally invasive direct coronary artery bypass improves late survival compared with drug-eluting stents in isolated proximal left anterior descending artery disease: a 10-year follow-up, single-center, propensity score analysis. *J Thorac Cardiovasc Surg*, 2014. 148(4): p. 1316-1322.

[18] Bonatti, J., Schachner, T., Bonaros, N. et al., Robotic totally endoscopic double-vessel bypass grafting: a further step toward closed-chest surgical treatment of multivessel coronary artery disease. *Heart Surg Forum*, 2007. 10(3): p. E239-242.

[19] Hillis, L.D., Smith, P.K., Anderson, J.L. et al., 2011 ACCF/AHA Guideline for Coronary Artery Bypass Graft Surgery. A report of the American College of Cardiology Foundation/American Heart Association Task Force on Practice Guidelines. Developed in collaboration with the American Association for Thoracic Surgery, Society of Cardiovascular Anesthesiologists, and Society of Thoracic Surgeons. *J Am Coll Cardiol*, 2011. 58(24): p. e123-210.

[20] Hillis, L.D., Smith, P.K., Anderson, J.L. et al., 2011 ACCF/AHA guideline for coronary artery bypass graft surgery: executive summary: a report of the American College of Cardiology Foundation/American Heart Association Task Force on Practice Guidelines. *J Thorac Cardiovasc Surg*, 2012. 143(1): p. 4-34.
[21] Fiore, A.C., Naunheim, K.S., Dean, P. et al., Results of internal thoracic artery grafting over 15 years: single versus double grafts. *Ann Thorac Surg*, 1990. 49(2): p. 202-208; discussion 208-209.
[22] Goldman, S., Zadina, K., Moritz, T. et al., Long-term patency of saphenous vein and left internal mammary artery grafts after coronary artery bypass surgery: results from a Department of Veterans Affairs Cooperative Study. *J Am Coll Cardiol*, 2004. 44(11): p. 2149-2156.
[23] Cheng, Y.T., Yu, J.B., Sun, T. et al., Ten years patency of left internal mammary artery trunk dissection graft after coronary artery bypass procedure. *Chin Med J* (Engl.), 2010. 123(22): p. 3354-3355.
[24] Kay, H.R., Korns, M.E., Flemma, R.J. et al., Atherosclerosis of the internal mammary artery. *Ann Thorac Surg*, 1976. 21(6): p. 504-507.
[25] Cheng, K., Rehman, S.M., and Taggart, D.P., A Review of Differing Techniques of Mammary Artery Harvesting on Sternal Perfusion: Time for a Randomized Study? *Ann Thorac Surg*, 2015. 100(5): p. 1942-1953.
[26] Boodhwani, M., Lam, B.K., Nathan, H.J. et al., Skeletonized internal thoracic artery harvest reduces pain and dysesthesia and improves sternal perfusion after coronary artery bypass surgery: a randomized, double-blind, within-patient comparison. *Circulation*, 2006. 114(8): p. 766-773.
[27] Harskamp, R.E., Alexander, J.H., Ferguson, T.B., Jr. et al., Frequency and Predictors of Internal Mammary Artery Graft Failure and Subsequent Clinical Outcomes: Insights From the PREVENT IV Trial. *Circulation*, 2015.
[28] Grau, J.B., Ferrari, G., Mak, A.W. et al., Propensity matched analysis of bilateral internal mammary artery versus single left internal mammary artery grafting at 17-year follow-up: validation of a contemporary surgical experience. *Eur J Cardiothorac Surg*, 2012. 41(4): p. 770-775; discussion 776.
[29] Vallely, M.P., Edelman, J.J., and Wilson, M.K., Bilateral internal mammary arteries: evidence and technical considerations. *Ann Cardiothorac Surg*, 2013. 2(4): p. 570-577.
[30] Davierwala, P.M. and Mohr, F.W., Bilateral internal mammary artery grafting: rationale and evidence. *Int J Surg*, 2015. 16(Pt B): p. 133-139.

[31] Yi, G., Shine, B., Rehman, S.M. et al., Effect of bilateral internal mammary artery grafts on long-term survival: a meta-analysis approach. *Circulation*, 2014. 130(7): p. 539-545.
[32] Weiss, A.J., Zhao, S., Tian, D.H. et al., A meta-analysis comparing bilateral internal mammary artery with left internal mammary artery for coronary artery bypass grafting. *Ann Cardiothorac Surg*, 2013. 2(4): p. 390-400.
[33] Harskamp, R.E., Lopes, R.D., Baisden, C.E. et al., Saphenous vein graft failure after coronary artery bypass surgery: pathophysiology, management, and future directions. *Ann Surg*, 2013. 257(5): p. 824-833.
[34] Harskamp, R.E., Alexander, J.H., Schulte, P.J. et al., Vein graft preservation solutions, patency, and outcomes after coronary artery bypass graft surgery: follow-up from the PREVENT IV randomized clinical trial. *JAMA Surg*, 2014. 149(8): p. 798-805.
[35] Zhang, H., Wang, Z.W., Wu, H.B. et al., Radial artery graft vs. saphenous vein graft for coronary artery bypass surgery : which conduit offers better efficacy? *Herz*, 2014. 39(4): p. 458-465.
[36] Bourassa, M.G., Fisher, L.D., Campeau, L. et al., Long-term fate of bypass grafts: the Coronary Artery Surgery Study (CASS) and Montreal Heart Institute experiences. *Circulation*, 1985. 72(6 Pt 2): p. V71-78.
[37] Rosch, J., Keller, F.S., and Kaufman, J.A., The birth, early years, and future of interventional radiology. *J Vasc Interv Radiol,* 2003. 14(7): p. 841-853.
[38] Meier, B., Bachmann, D., and Luscher, T., 25 years of coronary angioplasty: almost a fairy tale. *Lancet*, 2003. 361(9356): p. 527.
[39] Dotter, C.T. and Judkins, M.P., Transluminal Treatment Of Arteriosclerotic Obstruction. Description Of A New Technic And A Preliminary Report Of Its Application. *Circulation*, 1964. 30: p. 654-670.
[40] Morice, M.C., Serruys, P.W., Sousa, J.E. et al., A randomized comparison of a sirolimus-eluting stent with a standard stent for coronary revascularization. *N Engl J Med*, 2002. 346(23): p. 1773-1780.
[41] Ong, A.T., van Domburg, R.T., Aoki, J. et al., Sirolimus-eluting stents remain superior to bare-metal stents at two years: medium-term results from the Rapamycin-Eluting Stent Evaluated at Rotterdam Cardiology Hospital (RESEARCH) registry. *J Am Coll Cardiol*, 2006. 47(7): p. 1356-1360.
[42] Fajadet, J., Wijns, W., Laarman, G.J. et al., Randomized, double-blind, multicenter study of the Endeavor zotarolimus-eluting

phosphorylcholine-encapsulated stent for treatment of native coronary artery lesions: clinical and angiographic results of the ENDEAVOR II trial. *Circulation*, 2006. 114(8): p. 798-806.

[43] Serruys, P.W., Degertekin, M., Tanabe, K. et al., Intravascular ultrasound findings in the multicenter, randomized, double-blind RAVEL (RAndomized study with the sirolimus-eluting VElocity balloon-expandable stent in the treatment of patients with de novo native coronary artery Lesions) trial. *Circulation*, 2002. 106(7): p. 798-803.

[44] Serruys, P.W., Ong, A.T., Piek, J.J. et al., A randomized comparison of a durable polymer Everolimus-eluting stent with a bare metal coronary stent: The SPIRIT first trial. *EuroIntervention*, 2005. 1(1): p. 58-65.

[45] Palmerini, T., Biondi-Zoccai, G., Della Riva, D. et al., Stent thrombosis with drug-eluting and bare-metal stents: evidence from a comprehensive network meta-analysis. *Lancet*, 2012. 379(9824): p. 1393-1402.

[46] Ellis, S.G., Stone, G.W., Cox, D.A. et al., Long-term safety and efficacy with paclitaxel-eluting stents: 5-year final results of the TAXUS IV clinical trial (TAXUS IV-SR: Treatment of De Novo Coronary Disease Using a Single Paclitaxel-Eluting Stent). *JACC Cardiovasc Interv*, 2009. 2(12): p. 1248-1259.

[47] Weisz, G., Leon, M.B., Holmes, D.R., Jr. et al., Five-year follow-up after sirolimus-eluting stent implantation results of the SIRIUS (Sirolimus-Eluting Stent in De-Novo Native Coronary Lesions) Trial. *J Am Coll Cardiol*, 2009. 53(17): p. 1488-1497.

[48] Grines, C.L., Bonow, R.O., Casey, D.E., Jr. et al., Prevention of premature discontinuation of dual antiplatelet therapy in patients with coronary artery stents: a science advisory from the American Heart Association, American College of Cardiology, Society for Cardiovascular Angiography and Interventions, American College of Surgeons, and American Dental Association, with representation from the American College of Physicians. *J Am Dent Assoc*, 2007. 138(5): p. 652-655.

[49] Grines, C. and Cho, L., Atherothrombotic disease and the role of antiplatelet therapy in women. *J Womens Health* (Larchmt), 2008. 17(1): p. 35-46.

[50] Levine, G.N., Bates, E.R., Blankenship, J.C. et al., 2011 ACCF/AHA/ SCAI Guideline for Percutaneous Coronary Intervention: a report of the American College of Cardiology Foundation/American Heart Association Task Force on Practice Guidelines and the Society for

Cardiovascular Angiography and Interventions. *Circulation*, 2011. 124 (23): p. e574-651.

[51] Metzler, B. and Winkler, B., SYNTAX, STS and EuroSCORE - how good are they for risk estimation in atherosclerotic heart disease? *Thromb Haemost*, 2012. 108(6): p. 1065-1071.

[52] He, J.Q., Gao, Y.C., Yu, X.P. et al., Syntax score predicts clinical outcome in patients with three-vessel coronary artery disease undergoing percutaneous coronary intervention. *Chin Med J* (Engl), 2011. 124(5): p. 704-709.

[53] Sianos, G., Morel, M.A., Kappetein, A.P. et al., The SYNTAX Score: an angiographic tool grading the complexity of coronary artery disease. *EuroIntervention*, 2005. 1(2): p. 219-227.

[54] Serruys, P.W., Onuma, Y., Garg, S. et al., Assessment of the SYNTAX score in the Syntax study. *EuroIntervention*, 2009. 5(1): p. 50-56.

[55] Nam, C.W., Mangiacapra, F., Entjes, R. et al., Functional SYNTAX score for risk assessment in multivessel coronary artery disease. *J Am Coll Cardiol*, 2011. 58(12): p. 1211-1218.

[56] Farooq, V., Girasis, C., Magro, M. et al., The coronary artery bypass graft SYNTAX Score: final five-year outcomes from the SYNTAX-LE MANS left main angiographic substudy. *EuroIntervention*, 2013. 9(8): p. 1009-1010.

[57] Farooq, V., Head, S.J., Kappetein, A.P. et al., Widening clinical applications of the SYNTAX Score. *Heart*, 2014. 100(4): p. 276-287.

[58] Farooq, V., Serruys, P.W., Bourantas, C.V. et al., Quantification of incomplete revascularization and its association with five-year mortality in the synergy between percutaneous coronary intervention with taxus and cardiac surgery (SYNTAX) trial validation of the residual SYNTAX score. *Circulation*, 2013. 128(2): p. 141-151.

[59] Farooq, V., van Klaveren, D., Steyerberg, E.W. et al., Anatomical and clinical characteristics to guide decision making between coronary artery bypass surgery and percutaneous coronary intervention for individual patients: development and validation of SYNTAX score II. *Lancet*, 2013. 381(9867): p. 639-650.

[60] Nashef, S.A., Roques, F., Hammill, B.G. et al., Validation of European System for Cardiac Operative Risk Evaluation (EuroSCORE) in North American cardiac surgery. *Eur J Cardiothorac Surg*, 2002. 22(1): p. 101-105.

[61] Nashef, S.A., Roques, F., Michel, P. et al., European system for cardiac operative risk evaluation (EuroSCORE). *Eur J Cardiothorac Surg*, 1999. 16(1): p. 9-13.

[62] Nashef, S.A., Roques, F., Sharples, L.D. et al., EuroSCORE II. *Eur J Cardiothorac Surg,* 2012. 41(4): p. 734-744; discussion 744-735.

[63] The Society of Thoracic Surgeons. *Executive Summary: Society of Thoracic Surgeons Spring 2007 Report.* Chicago, IL: The Society of Thoracic Surgeons; 2007

[64] Kuwaki, K., Inaba, H., Yamamoto, T. et al., Performance of the EuroSCORE II and the Society of Thoracic Surgeons Score in patients undergoing aortic valve replacement for aortic stenosis. *J Cardiovasc Surg (Torino),* 2015. 56(3): p. 455-462.

[65] Loop, F.D., Lytle, B.W., Cosgrove, D.M. et al., Influence of the internal-mammary-artery graft on 10-year survival and other cardiac events. *N Engl J Med*, 1986. 314(1): p. 1-6.

[66] Smith, P.K., Califf, R.M., Tuttle, R.H. et al., Selection of surgical or percutaneous coronary intervention provides differential longevity benefit. *Ann Thorac Surg*, 2006. 82(4): p. 1420-1428; discussion 1428-1429.

[67] Greenbaum, A.B., Califf, R.M., Jones, R.H. et al., Comparison of medicine alone, coronary angioplasty, and left internal mammary artery-coronary artery bypass for one-vessel proximal left anterior descending coronary artery disease. *Am J Cardiol*, 2000. 86(12): p. 1322-1326.

[68] Diegeler, A., Thiele, H., Falk, V. et al., Comparison of stenting with minimally invasive bypass surgery for stenosis of the left anterior descending coronary artery. *N Engl J Med,* 2002. 347(8): p. 561-566.

[69] Harskamp, R.E., Williams, J.B., Halkos, M.E. et al., Meta-analysis of minimally invasive coronary artery bypass versus drug-eluting stents for isolated left anterior descending coronary artery disease (1097-685X (Electronic)).

[70] Taggart, D.P., Kaul, S., Boden, W.E. et al., Revascularization for unprotected left main stem coronary artery stenosis stenting or surgery. *J Am Coll Cardiol,* 2008. 51(9): p. 885-892.

[71] Harskamp, R.E. and Park, D.W., Stenting versus surgery for significant left main disease. *Curr Cardiol Rep*, 2015. 17(4): p. 18.

[72] Ahn, J.M., Roh, J.H., Kim, Y.H. et al., Randomized Trial of Stents Versus Bypass Surgery for Left Main Coronary Artery Disease: 5-Year Outcomes of the PRECOMBAT Study. *J Am Coll Cardiol*, 2015. 65 (20): p. 2198-2206.

[73] Harskamp, R.E. and Park, D.-W., Stenting Versus Surgery for Significant Left Main Disease. *Current Cardiology Reports*, 2015. 17 (4): p. 1-7.

[74] Levine, G.N., Bates, E.R., Blankenship, J.C. et al., 2011 ACCF/AHA/ SCAI guideline for percutaneous coronary intervention: a report of the American College of Cardiology Foundation/American Heart Association Task Force on Practice Guidelines and the Society for Cardiovascular Angiography and Interventions. *Catheter Cardiovasc Interv*, 2013. 82(4): p. E266-355.

[75] Buszman, P.E., Buszman, P.P., Kiesz, R.S. et al., Early and long-term results of unprotected left main coronary artery stenting: the LE MANS (Left Main Coronary Artery Stenting) registry. *J Am Coll Cardiol*, 2009. 54(16): p. 1500-1511.

[76] Park, S.J., Kim, Y.H., Park, D.W. et al., Randomized trial of stents versus bypass surgery for left main coronary artery disease. *N Engl J Med*, 2011. 364(18): p. 1718-1727.

[77] Boudriot, E., Thiele, H., Walther, T. et al., Randomized comparison of percutaneous coronary intervention with sirolimus-eluting stents versus coronary artery bypass grafting in unprotected left main stem stenosis. *J Am Coll Cardiol*, 2011. 57(5): p. 538-545.

[78] Morice, M.C., Serruys, P.W., Kappetein, A.P. et al., Outcomes in patients with de novo left main disease treated with either percutaneous coronary intervention using paclitaxel-eluting stents or coronary artery bypass graft treatment in the Synergy Between Percutaneous Coronary Intervention with TAXUS and Cardiac Surgery (SYNTAX) trial. *Circulation*, 2010. 121(24): p. 2645-2653.

[79] Mohr, F.W., Morice, M.C., Kappetein, A.P. et al., Coronary artery bypass graft surgery versus percutaneous coronary intervention in patients with three-vessel disease and left main coronary disease: 5-year follow-up of the randomised, clinical SYNTAX trial. *Lancet*, 2013. 381 (9867): p. 629-638.

[80] Buszman, P.E., Buszman, P.P., Banasiewicz-Szkrobka, I. et al., Left Main Stenting in Comparison With Surgical Revascularization: 10-Year Outcomes of the (Left Main Coronary Artery Stenting) LE MANS Trial. *JACC Cardiovasc Interv*, 2016. 9(4): p. 318-327.

[81] Corpus, R.A., House, J.A., Marso, S.P. et al., Multivessel percutaneous coronary intervention in patients with multivessel disease and acute myocardial infarction. *Am Heart J*, 2004. 148(3): p. 493-500.

[82] Boden, W.E., O'Rourke, R.A., Teo, K.K. et al., Optimal medical therapy with or without PCI for stable coronary disease. *N Engl J Med*, 2007. 356(15): p. 1503-1516.
[83] <Meta-analysis of 5-year outcomes of CABG vs PCI with stenting in patients with multivessel disease - PubMed Health.pdf>.
[84] Verma, S., Farkouh, M.E., Yanagawa, B. et al., Comparison of coronary artery bypass surgery and percutaneous coronary intervention in patients with diabetes: a meta-analysis of randomised controlled trials. *Lancet Diabetes Endocrinol*, 2013. 1(4): p. 317-328.
[85] Daemen, J., Boersma, E., Flather, M. et al., Long-term safety and efficacy of percutaneous coronary intervention with stenting and coronary artery bypass surgery for multivessel coronary artery disease: a meta-analysis with 5-year patient-level data from the ARTS, ERACI-II, MASS-II, and SoS trials. *Circulation*, 2008. 118(11): p. 1146-1154.
[86] Aggarwal, B., Goel, S.S., Sabik, J.F. et al., The FREEDOM trial: in appropriate patients with diabetes and multivessel coronary artery disease, CABG beats PCI. *Cleve Clin J Med*, 2013. 80(8): p. 515-523.
[87] Booth, J., Clayton, T., Pepper, J. et al., Randomized, controlled trial of coronary artery bypass surgery versus percutaneous coronary intervention in patients with multivessel coronary artery disease: six-year follow-up from the Stent or Surgery Trial (SoS). *Circulation*, 2008. 118(4): p. 381-388.
[88] Singh, M., Peterson, E.D., Roe, M.T. et al., Trends in the association between age and in-hospital mortality after percutaneous coronary intervention: National Cardiovascular Data Registry experience. *Circ Cardiovasc Interv*, 2009. 2(1): p. 20-26.
[89] Cohen, D.J., Van Hout, B., Serruys, P.W. et al., Quality of life after PCI with drug-eluting stents or coronary-artery bypass surgery. *N Engl J Med*, 2011. 364(11): p. 1016-1026.
[90] Zhang, Z., Kolm, P., Grau-Sepulveda, M.V. et al., Cost-effectiveness of revascularization strategies: the ASCERT study. *J Am Coll Cardiol*, 2015. 65(1): p. 1-11.
[91] Bangalore, S., Guo, Y., Samadashvili, Z. et al., Everolimus-eluting stents or bypass surgery for multivessel coronary disease. *N Engl J Med*, 2015. 372(13): p. 1213-1222.
[92] Investigators, B., The final 10-year follow-up results from the BARI randomized trial. *J Am Coll Cardiol*, 2007. 49(15): p. 1600-1606.
[93] Hueb, W., Lopes, N., Gersh, B.J. et al., Ten-year follow-up survival of the Medicine, Angioplasty, or Surgery Study (MASS II): a randomized

controlled clinical trial of 3 therapeutic strategies for multivessel coronary artery disease. *Circulation*, 2010. 122(10): p. 949-957.

[94] Park, S.J., Ahn, J.M., Kim, Y.H. et al., Trial of everolimus-eluting stents or bypass surgery for coronary disease. *N Engl J Med*, 2015. 372(13): p. 1204-1212.

[95] Bangalore, S., Blecker, S., and Hannan, E.L., Everolimus-Eluting Stents or Bypass Surgery for Coronary Disease. *N Engl J Med*, 2015. 373(6): p. 582.

[96] Bangalore, S., Guo, Y., Samadashvili, Z. et al., Revascularization in Patients With Multivessel Coronary Artery Disease and Chronic Kidney Disease: Everolimus-Eluting Stents Versus Coronary Artery Bypass Graft Surgery. *J Am Coll Cardiol*, 2015. 66(11): p. 1209-1220.

[97] Hochholzer, W., Buettner, H.J., Trenk, D. et al., Percutaneous coronary intervention versus coronary artery bypass grafting as primary revascularization in patients with acute coronary syndrome. *Am J Cardiol*, 2008. 102(2): p. 173-179.

[98] Fox, K.A., Poole-Wilson, P.A., Henderson, R.A. et al., Interventional versus conservative treatment for patients with unstable angina or non-ST-elevation myocardial infarction: the British Heart Foundation RITA 3 randomised trial. Randomized Intervention Trial of unstable Angina. *Lancet*, 2002. 360(9335): p. 743-751.

[99] Ben-Gal, Y., Weisz, G., Collins, M.B. et al., Dual catheter technique for the treatment of severe coronary artery perforations. *Catheter Cardiovasc Interv*, 2010. 75(5): p. 708-712.

[100] Weintraub, W.S., Grau-Sepulveda, M.V., Weiss, J.M. et al., Comparative effectiveness of revascularization strategies. *N Engl J Med*, 2012. 366(16): p. 1467-1476.

[101] Hlatky, M.A., Boothroyd, D.B., Bravata, D.M. et al., Coronary artery bypass surgery compared with percutaneous coronary interventions for multivessel disease: a collaborative analysis of individual patient data from ten randomised trials. *Lancet*, 2009. 373(9670): p. 1190-1197.

[102] Chieffo, A., Hoye, A., Mauri, F. et al., Gender-based issues in interventional cardiology: a consensus statement from the Women in Innovations (WIN) Initiative. *Catheter Cardiovasc Interv*, 2010. 75(2): p. 145-152.

[103] Guru, V., Fremes, S.E., Austin, P.C. et al., Gender differences in outcomes after hospital discharge from coronary artery bypass grafting. *Circulation*, 2006. 113(4): p. 507-516.

[104] Lempereur, M., Magne, J., Cornelis, K. et al., Impact of gender difference in hospital outcomes following percutaneous coronary intervention. Results of the Belgian Working Group on Interventional Cardiology (BWGIC) registry. *EuroIntervention*, 2014.
[105] Kornowski, R., Vaknin-Assa, H., Assali, A. et al., A comparative analysis of major clinical outcomes with drug-eluting stents versus bare metal stents in male versus female patients. *EuroIntervention*, 2012. 7 (9): p. 1051-1059.
[106] Brener, S.J., Lytle, B.W., Casserly, I.P. et al., Predictors of revascularization method and long-term outcome of percutaneous coronary intervention or repeat coronary bypass surgery in patients with multivessel coronary disease and previous coronary bypass surgery. *Eur Heart J*, 2006. 27(4): p. 413-418.
[107] Weintraub, W.S., Jones, E.L., Morris, D.C. et al., Outcome of reoperative coronary bypass surgery versus coronary angioplasty after previous bypass surgery. *Circulation*, 1997. 95(4): p. 868-877.
[108] Stephan, W.J., O'Keefe, J.H., Jr., Piehler, J.M. et al., Coronary angioplasty versus repeat coronary artery bypass grafting for patients with previous bypass surgery. *J Am Coll Cardiol*, 1996. 28(5): p. 1140-1146.
[109] Harskamp, R.E., Beijk, M.A., Damman, P. et al., Clinical outcome after surgical or percutaneous revascularization in coronary bypass graft failure. *J Cardiovasc Med* (Hagerstown), 2013. 14(6): p. 438-445.
[110] Hage, F.G., Venkataraman, R., Zoghbi, G.J. et al., The scope of coronary heart disease in patients with chronic kidney disease. *J Am Coll Cardiol*, 2009. 53(23): p. 2129-2140.
[111] Ashrith, G., Elayda, M.A., and Wilson, J.M., Revascularization options in patients with chronic kidney disease. *Tex Heart Inst J*, 2010. 37(1): p. 9-18.
[112] Bejan-Angoulvant, T., Bergerot, C., Juillard, L. et al., Myocardial microvascular disease and major adverse cardiovascular events in patients with end-stage renal disease: rationale and design of the MICROCARD study. *Nephrol Dial Transplant*, 2012. 27(7): p. 2886-2891.
[113] Sharma, S., Farrington, K., Kozarski, R. et al., Impaired thrombolysis: a novel cardiovascular risk factor in end-stage renal disease. *Eur Heart J*, 2013. 34(5): p. 354-363.

[114] Hemmelgarn, B.R., Southern, D., Culleton, B.F. et al., Survival after coronary revascularization among patients with kidney disease. *Circulation*, 2004. 110(14): p. 1890-1895.
[115] Krishnaswami, A., McCulloch, C.E., Tawadrous, M. et al., Coronary artery bypass grafting and percutaneous coronary intervention in patients with end-stage renal disease. *Eur J Cardiothorac Surg*, 2015. 47(5): p. e193-198.
[116] Gupta, T., Harikrishnan, P., Kolte, D. et al., Trends in management and outcomes of ST-elevation myocardial infarction in patients with end-stage renal disease in the United States. *Am J Cardiol*, 2015. 115(8): p. 1033-1041.
[117] Farkouh, M.E., Domanski, M., Sleeper, L.A. et al., Strategies for multivessel revascularization in patients with diabetes. *N Engl J Med*, 2012. 367(25): p. 2375-2384.
[118] Dangas, G.D., Farkouh, M.E., Sleeper, L.A. et al., Long-term outcome of PCI versus CABG in insulin and non-insulin-treated diabetic patients: results from the FREEDOM trial. *J Am Coll Cardiol*, 2014. 64(12): p. 1189-1197.
[119] Kapur, A., Hall, R.J., Malik, I.S. et al., Randomized comparison of percutaneous coronary intervention with coronary artery bypass grafting in diabetic patients. 1-year results of the CARDia (Coronary Artery Revascularization in Diabetes) trial. *J Am Coll Cardiol*, 2010. 55(5): p. 432-440.
[120] Farkouh, M.E., Domanski, M., Sleeper, L.A. et al., Strategies for multivessel revascularization in patients with diabetes. *N Engl J Med*, 2012. 367(25): p. 2375-2384.
[121] Kappetein, A.P., Head, S.J., Morice, M.C. et al., Treatment of complex coronary artery disease in patients with diabetes: 5-year results comparing outcomes of bypass surgery and percutaneous coronary intervention in the SYNTAX trial. *Eur J Cardiothorac Surg,* 2013. 43 (5): p. 1006-1013.
[122] Kamalesh, M., Sharp, T.G., Tang, X.C. et al., Percutaneous coronary intervention versus coronary bypass surgery in United States veterans with diabetes. *J Am Coll Cardiol*, 2013. 61(8): p. 808-816.
[123] Williams, J.B., Harskamp, R.E., Bose, S. et al., The Preservation and Handling of Vein Grafts in Current Surgical Practice: Findings of a Survey Among Cardiovascular Surgeons of Top-Ranked US Hospitals. *JAMA Surg*, 2015. 150(7): p. 681-683.

[124] Harskamp, R.E., Vassiliades, T.A., Mehta, R.H. et al., Comparative Effectiveness of Hybrid Coronary Revascularization vs Coronary Artery Bypass Grafting. *J Am Coll Surg*, 2015. 221(2): p. 326-334 e321.

[125] Harskamp, R.E., Halkos, M.E., Xian, Y. et al., A nationwide survey on perception, experience, and expectations of hybrid coronary revascularization among top-ranked US hospitals. *Am Heart J*, 2015. 169(4): p. 557-563 e556.

[126] Kern, M.J. and Samady, H., Current concepts of integrated coronary physiology in the catheterization laboratory. *J Am Coll Cardiol*, 2010. 55(3): p. 173-185.

[127] Tonino, P.A., De Bruyne, B., Pijls, N.H. et al., Fractional flow reserve versus angiography for guiding percutaneous coronary intervention. *N Engl J Med*, 2009. 360(3): p. 213-224.

Biographical Sketch

Name: Sameer Hirji

Affiliation: Department of Surgery, Brigham and Women's Hospital, Harvard Medical School

Duke Clinical Research Institute

Education: Massachusetts Institute of Technology (MIT) (B.S.)

Duke University School of Medicine (MD)

Harvard Medical School (M.D. Candidate)

Experience: My research experience is mainly in the field of general and cardiothoracic surgery, with specific interest in optimizing outcomes of patients undergoing cardiac surgery, heart and lung transplantation. My research particularly focuses on large databases and registries, with a goal of performing comparative effective analysis and developing risk prediction models.

Honors:

2014 James W. Brooks Scholarship Finalist (Southern Thoracic Surgical Association, (STSA); Poster Distinction Award, World Transplant Congress, San Francisco, CA July 2013; American Association of Thoracic Surgeons (AATS) Summer Intern Scholarship in Cardiothoracic Surgery (2013)

Publications Last 3 Years:

1. Hirji SA, Balderson SS, Berry MF, D'Amico TA. Troubleshooting thoracoscopic anterior mediastinal surgery: lessons learned from

thoracoscopic lobectomy. *Ann Cardiothorac Surg*. 2015 Nov; 4(6): 545-9. PMID: 26693151.

2. Hirji SA, C Bravo, RE. Pachon, Anderson KL, MH. Sketch Jr., GD Sanders, E.M Ohman, SW. Zarich, JM Brennan. Early invasive versus conservative strategies for Non-Infarct Related Artery (non-IRA) lesions in ST Elevation Myocardial Infarction (STEMI) patients with Multi-vessel Disease. *Cochrane Review* 2015 Dec. 17; doi:10.1002/ 14651858.CD011986.
3. Gulack BC, Ganapathi AM, Speicher PJ, Meza JM, Hirji SA, Snyder LD, Davis RD, Hartwig MG. What Is the Optimal Transplant for Older Patients With Idiopathic Pulmonary Fibrosis? *Ann Thorac Surg*. 2015 Nov; 100(5):1826-33. PMID: 26210946; PMCID: PMC46301 42.
4. Ganapathi AM, Hirji SA, Wang A, Patel CB, Gaca JG, Schroder JN. Bridge to long-term mechanical circulatory support with a left ventricular assist device: novel use of transcatheter aortic valve replacement. *Ann Thorac Surg*. 2015 Apr; 99(4):e91-3. PMID: 25841 859.
5. Hirji SA, Haney JC, Welsby I, Lombard FW, Berry MF. Hyperbaric oxygen therapy for treatment of neurologic sequela after atrioesophageal fistula. *Ann Thorac Surg*. 2015 Feb; 99(2):681-2. PMID: 25639405.
6. Park DW, Clare RM, Schulte PJ, Pieper KS, Shaw LK, Califf RM, Ohman EM, Van de Werf F, Hirji S, Harrington RA, Armstrong PW, Granger CB, Jeong MH, Patel MR. Extent, location, and clinical significance of non-infarct-related coronary artery disease among patients with ST-elevation myocardial infarction. *JAMA*. 2014 Nov 19; 312(19):2019-27. PMID: 25399277.
7. Osho AA, Castleberry AW, Snyder LD, Palmer SM, Ganapathi AM, Hirji SA, Lin SS, Davis RD, Hartwig MG. Differential outcomes with early and late repeat transplantation in the era of the lung allocation score. *Ann Thorac Surg*. 2014 Dec; 98(6):1914-20; discussion 1920-1. PMID: 25442999.
8. Osho AA, Castleberry AW, Snyder LD, Ganapathi AM, Speicher PJ, Hirji SA, Stafford-Smith M, Daneshmand MA, Duane Davis R, Hartwig MG. Determining eligibility for lung transplantation: A nationwide assessment of the cutoff glomerular filtration rate. *J Heart Lung Transplant*. 2015 Apr; 34(4):571-9. PMID: 25524142.

9. Kara HV, Javidfar J, Hirji SA, Balderson SS, D'Amico TA. Thoracoscopic pneumonectomy in management of histoplasmosis and fibrosing mediastinitis. *Ann Thorac Surg*. 2014 Oct; 98(4):e95-6. PMID: 25282249.
10. Harskamp RE, Abdelsalam M, Lopes RD, Boga G, Hirji S, Krishnan M, Kiljanek L, Mumtaz M, Tijssen JG, McCarty C, de Winter RJ, Bachinsky WB. Cardiac troponin release following hybrid coronary revascularization versus off-pump coronary artery bypass surgery. *Interact Cardiovasc Thorac Surg*. 2014 Dec; 19(6):1008-12. PMID: 25217621.
11. Speicher PJ, Ganapathi AM, Englum BR, Gulack BC, Osho AA, Hirji SA, Castleberry AW, Snyder LD, Duane Davis R, Hartwig MG. Single-lung transplantation in the United States: what happens to the other lung? *J Heart Lung Transplant*. 2015 Jan; 34(1):36-42. PMID: 25305097; PMCID: PMC4339113.
12. Gulack BC, Hirji SA, Hartwig MG. Bridge to lung transplantation and rescue post-transplant: the expanding role of extracorporeal membrane oxygenation. *J Thorac Dis*. 2014 Aug; 6(8):1070-9. PMID: 25132974; PMCID: PMC4133542.
13. Osho AA, Castleberry AW, Snyder LD, Ganapathi AM, Hirji SA, Stafford-Smith M, Lin SS, Davis RD, Hartwig MG. Assessment of different threshold preoperative glomerular filtration rates as markers of outcomes in lung transplantation. *Ann Thorac Surg*. 2014 Jul; 98 (1):283-9; discussion 289-90. PMID: 24793682; PMCID: PMC4332517.
14. Klapper J, Hirji S, Hartwig MG, D'Amico TA, Harpole DH, Onaitis MW, Berry MF. Outcomes after pneumonectomy for benign disease: the impact of urgent resection. *J Am Coll Surg*. 2014 Sep; 219(3):518-24. PMID: 24862885; PMCID: PMC4143430.

Name: Faith C. Robertson

Affiliation: Harvard Medical School

Brigham and Women's Hospital

Education: Duke University. Durham, NC. (B.S.)

National Cancer Institute, National Institutes of Health (Research Fellowship)

Harvard Medical School (M.D. Candidate)

Experience: My research experience is mainly in the field of general surgery and oncology, with particular interest in public health and quality improvement practices.

Honors:

Graduation with High Distinction, Duke University, 2013

Cancer Research Trainee Award, National Institutes of Health, 2013-2014

Outstanding Poster Award, NIH Postbac Poster Day, 2014

Publications Last 3 Years:

1. Robertson FC, Berzofsky JA, Terabe M. Nkt cell networks in the regulation of tumor immunity. *Front Immunol*. 2014;5:3389.
2. Spector NL, Robertson FC, Bacus S, Blackwell K, Smith DA, Glenn K et al. Lapatinib plasma and tumor concentrations and effects on her receptor phosphorylation in tumor. *PloS one*. 2015;10:e0142845.

Name: Kevin L Anderson, Jr.

Affiliation: Duke University School of Medicine

Education: B.S., Morehouse College

Publications Last 3 Years:

1. Yang CF, Meyerhoff RR, Stephens SJ, Singhapricha T, Toomey CB, Anderson KL, Kelsey C, Harpole D, D'Amico TA, Berry MF. Long-term outcomes of lobectomy for non-small cell lung cancer after definitive radiation treatment. *Ann Thorac Surg. 2015 Apr. 15*. pii: S0003-4975(15)00215-5. doi: 10.1016/j.athoracsur.2015.01.064.
2. Yang CF, Adil SM, Anderson KL, Meyerhoff RR, Hartwig MG, Harpole DH, Tong BC, Berry MF. Impact of patient selection and treatment strategies on outcomes after lobectomy for biopsy-proven stage IIIA pN2 non-small cell lung cancer. *Eur J Cardiothorac Surg* 2015 Dec 30. doi: 10.1093/ejcts/ezv431.
3. Hirji SA, C Bravo, RE. Pachon, Anderson KL, MH. Sketch Jr., GD Sanders, E.M Ohman, SW. Zarich, JM Brennan. Early invasive versus conservative strategies for Non-Infarct Related Artery (non-IRA) lesions in ST Elevation Myocardial Infarction (STEMI) patients with Multi-vessel Disease. *Cochrane Review* 2015 Dec 17; doi:10.1002/ 14651858.CD011986.

Name: Ralf E Harskamp

Affiliation: University of Amsterdam

Education: University of Groningen (MD), with internships at the University of Pennsylvania and University of Texas

University of Amsterdam (PhD)

Duke University (research fellowship)

Experience: My research experience is mainly in the field of clinical medicine, with specific interest in improving care for patients with coronary artery disease. Over the past 5 years this has resulted in collaborations with front runners in the field of cardiovascular medicine, such as Duke University and Emory University.

Professional Appointments: Research fellow at the University of Amsterdam

Honors: Best Fellow In Training Poster Award – American College of Cardiology Scientific Sessions, San Francisco, CA, March 2013

Publications Last 3 Years:

1. Harskamp RE, Clare RM, Ambrosio G, Held C, Lokhnygina Y, Moliterno DJ, White HD, Aylward PE, Armstrong PW, Mahaffey KW, Harrington RA, Van de Werf F, Wallentin L, Strony J, Tricoci P. Use of thienopyridine prior to presentation for non-ST-segment elevation acute coronary syndromes and association with safety and efficacy of Vorapaxar: insights from the TRACER trial. *Eur Heart J Acute Cardiovasc Care* 2016 Feb; Accepted.
2. Sebben JC, Pinto Ribeiro DR, Lopes RD, de Winter RJ, Harskamp R, Cambruzzi E, Schmidt MM, Schutz Martinelli E, Gottschall CA, Quadros AS. The role of diabetes mellitus in the composion of coronary thrombi in patients presenting with acute ST-segment elevation myocardial infarction undergoing primary percutaneous coronary intervention. *Am Heart J* 2016;172:26-33.
3. Rosenblum JM, Harskamp RE, Hoedemaker N, Walker P, Liberman HA, de Winter RJ, Vassiliades TA, Puskas JD, Halkos ME. Hybrid coronary revascularization versus coronary artery bypass surgery with bilateral or single internal mammary artery grafts. *J Thorac Cardiovasc Surg* 2015 Oct. 26 Epub. ahead of print.
4. Harskamp RE, Alexander JH, Ferguson TB Jr, Hager R, Mack MJ, Englum B, Wojdyla D, Schulte PJ, Kouchoukos NT, de Winter RJ, Gibson CM, Peterson ED, Harrington RA, Smith PK, Lopes RD. Frequency and predictors of internal mammary artery graft failure and

subsequent clinical outcomes: insights from the PREVENT IV trial. *Circulation* 2016;133:131-138.
5. Harskamp RE, Hoedemaker N, Newby LK, Woudstra P, Grundeken MJ, Beijk MA, Piek JJ, Tijssen JG, Mehta RH, de Winter RJ. Procedural and clinical outcomes after use of the glycoprotein IIb/IIIa inhibitor abciximab for saphenous vein graft interventions. *Cardiovasc Revasc Med* 2015; Oct 31, Epub.
6. Harskamp RE. Current state and future direction of hybrid coronary revascularization. *Curr Opin Cardiol* 2015;30:643-9.
7. Harskamp RE, Vassiliades TA, Mehta RH, de Winter RJ, Lopes RD, Xian Y, Peterson ED, Puskas JD, Halkos ME. Comparative effectiveness of hybrid coronary revascularization vs coronary artery bypass grafting. *J Am Coll Surg* 2015;221;326-34.
8. Williams JB, Harskamp RE, Bose S, Lawson JH, Alexander JH, Smith PK, Lopes RD. The preservation and handling of vein grafts in current surgical practice: findings of a survey among cardiovascular surgeons of top-ranked US hospitals. *JAMA Surg* 2015;150:681-3.
9. Harskamp RE, Halkos ME, Xian Y, Szerlip MA, Poston RS, Mick SL, Lopes RD, Tijssen JG, de Winter RJ, Peterson ED. A nationwide survey on perception, experience, and expectations of hybrid coronary revascularization among top-ranked US hospitals. *Am Heart J* 2015; 169:557-63.
10. Harskamp RE, Park DW. Stenting versus surgery for signficant left main diseasse. *Curr Cardiol Rep* 2015;17:574-5.
11. Harskamp RE, Schulte PJ, Alexander JH, Lopes RD. Reply: About the impact of extracardiac vascular disease on vein graft failure. *Ann Thorac Surg* 2014;98:1890.
12. Harskamp RE, Roe MT. Soluble urokinase-type plasminogen activator receptor: a useful biomarker for coronary artery disease and clinical outcomes? *J Am Heart Assoc* 2014;3:e001431.
13. Harskamp RE, Walker PF, Alexander JH, Xian Y, Liberman HA, de Winter RJ, Vassiliades TA, Peterson ED, Puskas JD, Halkos ME. Clinical outcomes of hybrid coronary revascularization versus coronary artery bypass surgery in patients with diabetes mellitus. *Am Heart J* 2014;168:471-8.
14. Harskamp RE, Abdelsalam M, Lopes RD, Boga G, Hirji S, Krishnan M, Kiljanek L, Mumtaz M, Tijssen JG, McCarty C, de Winter RJ, Bachinsky WB. Cardiac troponin release following hybrid coronary

revascularization versus off-pump coronary artery bypass surgery. *Interact Cardiovasc Thorac Surg* 2014;19:1008-12.

15. Harskamp RE, Alexander JH, Schulte PJ, Brophy CM, Mack MJ, Peterson ED, Williams JB, Gibson CM, Califf RM, Kouchoukos NT, Harrington RA, Ferguson TB Jr, Lopes RD. Vein graft preservation solutions, patency, and outcomes after coronary artery bypass graft surgery: follow-up from the PREVENT-IV randomized clinical trial. *JAMA Surg* 2014;149:798-805.
16. Harskamp RE, Brennan JM, Xian Y, Halkos ME, Puskas JD, Thourani VH, Gammie JS, Taylor BS, de Winter RJ, Kim S, O'Brien S, Peterson ED, Gaca JG. Practice patterns and clinical outcomes after hybrid coronary revascularization in the United States: an analysis from the society of thoracic surgeons adult cardiac database. *Circulation* 2014:130:872-9.
17. Williams JB, Peterson ED, Wojdyla D, Harskamp RE, Southerland KW, Ferguson TB, Smith PK, Milano CA, Lopes RD. Central venous pressure after coronary artery bypass surgery: does it predict postoperative mortality or renal failure? *J Crit Care* 2014;29:1006-10.
18. Harskamp RE, Puskas JD, Tijssen JG, Walker PF, Liberman HA, Lopes RD, Vassiliades TA, Peterson ED, Halkos ME. Comparison of hybrid coronary revascularization versus coronary artery bypass grafting in patients ≥65 years with multivessel coronary artery disease. *Am J Cardiol* 2014;114:224-9.
19. Harskamp RE, Williams JB, Halkos ME, Lopes RD, Tijssen JG, Ferguson TB Jr., de Winter RJ. Meta-analysis of minimally invasive coronary artery bypass versus drug-eluting stents for isolated left anterior descending coronary artery disease. *J Thorac Cardiovasc Surg* 2014;148:1837-42.
20. Harskamp RE, Newby LK. ACP Journal Club: Review: CABG reduces long-term mortality and morbidity more than PCI in multivessel coronary artery disease. *Ann Intern Med* 2014:160:JC9.
21. Ohman EM, Harskamp RE. We need to do better for patients with non-ST-segment elevation acute coronary syndrome who are managed without revascularization. *J Am Coll Cardiol* 2014;63:2258-60.
22. Harskamp RE, Bagai A, Halkos ME, Rao SV, Bachinsky WB, Patel MR, de Winter RJ, Peterson ED, Alexander JH, Lopes RD. Clinical outcomes after hybrid coronary revascularization versus coronary artery bypass surgery: a meta-analysis of 1,190 patients. *Am Heart J* 2014;167:585-92.

23. Harskamp RE, Wang TY, Bhatt DL, Wiviott SD, Amsterdam EA, Li S, Thomas L, de Winter RJ, Roe MT. Hospital patterns of medical management strategy use for patients with non-ST-elevation myocardial infarction and 3-vessel or left main coronary artery disease. *Am Heart J* 2014;167:355-362.
24. Harskamp RE, Zheng Z, Alexander JH, Williams JB, Xian Y, Halkos ME, Brennan JM, de Winter RJ, Smith PK, Lopes RD. Status quo of hybrid coronary revascularization for multi-vessel coronary artery disease. *Ann Thorac Surg* 2013;96:2268-77.
25. Harskamp RE, Alexander JH, Schulte PJ, Jones WS, Williams JB, Mack MJ, Peterson ED, Gibson CM, Califf RM, Kouchoukos NT, Ferguson TB, de Winter RJ, Lopes RD. Impact of extracardiac vascular disease on vein graft failure and outcomes after coronary artery bypass surgery. *Ann Thorac Surg* 2014;97:824-30.
26. Harskamp RE, Bonatti JO, Zhao DX, Puskas JD, de Winter RJ, Alexander JH, Halkos ME. Standardizing definitions for hybrid coronary revascularization. *J Thorac Cardiovasc Surg* 2014;147:556-60.
27. Harskamp RE, Kuijt WJ, Damman P, Beijk MA, Grundeken MJ, Woudstra P, Tijssen JG, de Winter RJ. Percutaneous coronary intervention for acute coronary syndrome due to graft failure: use of bare-metal and drug-eluting stents and subsequent long-term clinical outcome. *Catheter Cardiovasc Interv* 2014;83:203-9.
28. Harskamp RE, Park DW. Optimal choice of coronary revascularization and stent type in diabetic patients with coronary artery disease. *Cardiol Ther* 2013;2:69-84.
29. Beijk MA, Harskamp RE. Treatment of coronary artery bypass graft failure. *Book chapter: "Artery Bypass,"* editor: WS Aronow. ISBN: 978-953-51-1025-5, published March 13, 2013.
30. Harskamp RE, Williams JB, Hill RC, de Winter RJ, Alexander JH, Lopes RD. Saphenous vein graft failure and clinical outcomes: toward a surrogate end point in patients following coronary artery bypass surgery? *Am Heart J* 2013;165:639-43.
31. Harskamp RE, Park DW. Percutaneous coronary intervention in diabetic patients: should choice of stents be influenced? *Expert Rev Cardiovasc Ther* 2013:11:541-53.
32. Harskamp RE, Lopes RD, Baisden CE, de Winter RJ, Alexander JH. Saphenous vein graft failure after coronary artery bypass surgery:

pathophysiology, management, and future directions. *Ann Surg* 2013; 257:824-33.
33. Harskamp RE, Beijk MA, Damman P, Tijssen JG, Lopes RD, de Winter RJ. Prehospitalization antiplatelet therapy and outcomes after saphenous vein graft intervention. *Am J Cardiol* 2013;111:153-8.
34. Damman P, Kampinga MA, van der Horst IC, Woudstra P, Grundeken MJ, Kuijt WJ, Harskamp RE, Nijsten MW, Zijlstra F, Tijssen JG, de Smet BJ, de Winter RJ. Multiple biomarkers for the prediction and short and long-term mortality after ST-segment elevation myocardial infarction: the Amsterdam Groningen collaboration. *J Thromb Thrombolysis* 2013;36:42-6.
35. Damman P, Woudstra P, Kuijt WJ, Kikkert WJ, van de Hoef TP, Grundeken MJ, Harskamp RE, Henriques JP, Piek JJ, Tijssen JG, de Winter RJ. Short- and long-term prognostic value of the TIMI risk score after primary percutaneous coronary intervention for ST-segment elevation myocardial infarction. *J Interv Cardiol* 2013;26:8-13.
36. Harskamp RE, Beijk MA, Damman P, Kuijt WJ, Woudstra P, Grundeken MJ, Kloek JJ, Tijssen JG, de Mol BA, de Winter RJ. Clinical outcome after surgical or percutaneous revascularization in coronary bypass graft failure. *J Cardiovasc Med* 2013;14:438-45.
37. Woudstra P, Damman P, Beijk MA, Grundeken MJ, Harskamp RE, Koch KT, Henriques JP, Baan J Jr, Vis MM, Piek JJ, Tijssen JG, de Winter RJ. Clinical outcomes after bare-metal stenting in diabetic patients with lesions carrying a low risk of restenosis. *Catheter Cardiovasc Interv* 2013;81:26-33.

In: Coronary Artery Disease
Editor: Courtney Burke

ISBN: 978-1-63485-330-9

Chapter 3

GENDER DISPARITY IN CARDIOVASCULAR DISEASE: CONTRIBUTING FACTS AND FABLES

Parloop A. Bhatt* and Akshita Bhatt
L. M. College of Pharmacy, Navrangpura, Ahmedabad, India

ABSTRACT

Cardiovascular disease (CVD) affects men and women equally. Yet CVD is considered as a "Man's Disease". The patho-physiology of CVD differs significantly between the sexes. Thus American College of Cardiology (2011) laid specific guidelines focusing on women specific CVD prevention, diagnosis, management, treatment and outcomes. Compared to men, women are under-prevented, under-diagnosed, under-treated and under-studied with respect to CVD. Although women share similar risk factors like age, hypertension, diabetes, hyperlipidemia, obesity, family history of CVD with men; women specific variables like depression, pre-eclampsia, gestational diabetes, thyroid disease, psoriasis, gout and auto immune disorders contribute significantly. Besides, inflammatory markers suggesting risk of disease like high sensitivity C reactive protein are higher in women at baseline then men. Estrogen and progesterone are more influential in women; menstruation can affect hematologic and electrocardiographic indices; women have reduced sympathetic and enhanced parasympathetic activity. In response to stress,

*Corresponding author: Email: parloop72@gmail.com.

women experience an increased pulse rate, resulting in an increased cardiac output; men result in increased vascular resistance resulting in increased blood pressure. Difference in pain perception exists between sexes, resulting in variability in presenting symptoms. Women are more likely to attribute their symptoms to non cardiac causes complicating timely treatment. Recent acute coronary syndrome registries have shown that on admission women are less likely to receive heparin, ACE inhibitors, glycoprotein IIa/IIIb inhibitors; at discharge less likely to be prescribed aspirin and statin therapy. Women experience more drug related adverse events than men. Many specific areas of CVD like heart failure, atrial fibrillation, valvular and structural disease, peripheral vascular and cerebro-vascular disease should be examined for existing gender differences.

The healthcare sector holds a very critical and contributing role in education of adult female subjects towards risks of CVD; women specific contributing factors; warning signs; strategies to avoid delay in treatment; promote adherence to lifestyle interventions; ensure proper dosage adjustments to reduce risk of bleeding and other adverse events; promote primary and secondary prevention guidelines; improve application of evidence based therapy to improve women care in CVD.

INTRODUCTION

Although considered as a "Man's Disease" and developing later as compared to men,Cardiovascular disease (CVD) has been the major cause of death in women over 65 years of age. Compared to men, women are under-prevented, under-diagnosed, under-treated and under-studied with respect to CVD.Thus American College of Cardiology(2011) laid specific guidelines focusing on women specific CVD prevention, diagnosis, management, treatment and outcomes[1]. This chapter highlights the contributing patho-physiological factors in women, discussing specific areas of CVD like heart failure, atrial fibrillation, and peripheral vascular disease for existing gender differences. The chapter concludes citing application of evidence based therapy to improve women care in CVD.

BIOLOGICAL PARAMETERS

The biological differences in response to CVD between men and women include smaller vessel size; left ventricular end-diastolic dimension; lower collateral flow and coronary reserve and atheroma burden with higher vascular stiffness and functional differences of smooth muscle cells in women [2-4]. There is 10 percent lower stroke volume in women and the pulse rate of women is 3-5 beats/minute faster [4]. Men have enhanced parasympathetic activity while women have enhanced sympathetic activity and vice versa. Under the conditions of stress, the cardiac output increases in women due to an increase in pulse rate and in men, there is an increase in blood pressure due to increased vascular resistance [5]. In women, the concentration of nor epinephrine in plasma, number of circulating red blood cells per unit volume of plasma, hemoglobin is in lower amount and hence is the oxygen carrying capacity as compared to men [5]. Their sensitivity to altitude or body positioning changes leads them to experience of orthostatic hypotension and syncope [5]. Hematologic and electrographic indices are affected by menstruation and the predominance of testosterone in men and estrogen in women also influence the response of the body towards various ailments. Estrogen acts as a cardio protective and an immune-modulator in the body [6]. As the estrogen levels reduce in women after menopause, the risk for developing CVD increases several folds [7].

RISK FACTORS

Traditional as well as emerging risk factors include lifestyle interventions, pharmacotherapy, or a combination of two [8]. Though men and women share the same risk factors overall, certain risk factors like hypertension, diabetes, dyslipidemia, depression, may exert greater overall risk in women.

Hypertension is more widespread among women more so in sixth decade than men; being more severe in African American descent than any other cultural group [9]. In women prehypertension (blood pressure of 130-139/84-89 mm Hg), is associated with a 2.5 higher cardiovascular death, myocardial infarction (MI), stroke, and heart failure risk whereas in men it presents a 1.6 greater risk of mortality [10].

Diabetes: In diabetic men risk of cardiovascular disease is two to three fold whereas in women it increases by three to seven times [11-15]. Insulin affects the cardio protective effect of estradiol by causing a change in vascular smooth muscle cell proliferation leading to atherosclerosis [16, 17, 18].

Dyslipidemia: Following menopause, LDL levels and total cholesterol levels significantly rise in women [19-22]. Higher triglyceride levels and low HDL levels in women are considered to be more significant to cause CVD whereas high LDL and total cholesterol levels in men are more significant biomarkers [23, 24]. According to Adult Treatment Panel (ATP), guidelines for the diagnosis of metabolic syndrome, HDL <50 mg/dL in women and <40mg/dL in men are considered as risk factor [25].

Depression: A psychosocial risk also contributes to the pathogenesis of CVD twice in women as compared to men [26, 27]. In an observational, single centre study performed between January 2010 and December 2011 in Ahmedabad, Gujarat, India, 1648 (39%)out of 6867 patients suffering from CAD were diagnosed with depression, being higher in women as assessed by MARDS scale [28].

Gout: A study comparing gout in men and women concluded that women suffering from gout are at 39 percent greater risk of getting a heart attack and 41 percent more likely of getting a non-fatal heart attack than those without the disease whereas the risk factor in men suffering from gout of getting a heart attack is 11 percent higher than those who are free from gout [29].

WOMEN SPECIFIC VARIABLES

Pre-eclampsia: Early onset of preeclampsia is directly linked with an increase in risk of CVD [30]. Patients of preeclampsia have a risk of developing chronic hypertension, ischemic heart disease and stroke, the risk being greater in those in whom the diagnosis is made before 37 weeks [31].

Gestational Diabetes: It is recognized that Gestational Diabetes Mellitus (GDM) increases the risk for developing type 2 diabetes mellitus (T2DM) [32],atherosclerosis and CVD [33-36].Studies reveal that women with GDM have an increased common carotid artery intima-media thickness [37].

Hormone Therapy: Menopause is accompanied by undesirable levels of CVD risk factors, which include alterations in body fat, distribution from gynoid to android pattern, increased plasma lipids, increase in sympathetic tone, dysfunctional endothelium, and hypertension [7]. Low levels of estrogens following menopause reduces vasomotor tone [38]. The overall effects of hormone therapy are totally dependent on the dose and type of estrogens, risk of CVD, ones' current age and age at menopause, cancer risks and family medical history [39, 40].

Thyroid Disease: Untreated hypothyroidism in women produces an increased total and LDL cholesterol. Unlike men, women with greater than 7mmol/L total cholesterol had a seven fold increased risk of hypothyroidism [41].

SPECIFIC CARDIOVASCULAR DISEASES IN WOMEN

Heart Failure in Women

Although nearly 50% of the female CVD mortality is due to CAD, 35% is due to heart failure (HF) [42].

Prevalence and Causes

Prevalence of HF increases with age, however more women than men have HF after 79 years of age [42]. From both the Framingham and the Olmstead County databases, more women than men have HF (diastolic) with preserved LV function [43, 44,45].Women with impaired LV systolic function tend to present with a higher left ventricular ejection fraction (LVEF) when compared with men [46]. Although, co-morbidities are common, hypertension, smoking and CAD are more contributing in women [47]. Prevalence of thyroid disease is more frequent in women with acute decompensated HF, whereas chronic obstructive lung disease, peripheral vascular disease, and renal insufficiency are more common in men [43, 46]. Other causes of HF in women include cardiac toxicity from chemotherapeutic agents used to treat breast malignancy and peripartum cardiomyopathy; other potential causes include myocarditis, abnormal immune response to pregnancy, increased myocyte apoptosis, genetic predisposition, and proteolytic cleavage of prolactin during oxidative stress. Preliminary data suggests usage of bromocriptine to suppress lactation in the post-partum period has been associated with increased incidence of cardiovascular events, hypertension, and thrombus formation [48]; other associated risk factors include advanced maternal age, African descent, high parity, twin pregnancy, usage of tocolytics, and poverty [48].

Diagnosis

Although diagnosis of HF is based on a constellation of symptoms and signs [49], according to SOLVD (Studies Of Left Ventricular Dysfunction) database, women with impaired systolic LV function are more likely than men to have dependent edema, jugular venous distension, and an S3 gallop [50]. In contrast, according to ADHERE (Acute Decompensated Heart Failure National Registry) (impaired and preserved systolic function), there were no clinically important differences in the frequency of HF symptoms/signs between women (n = 54,674) and men (n = 50,713) [43]. Biomarker brain natriuretic peptide values were higher in women versus men [51].

Treatment

ACEIs are currently recommended for all patients with HF and impaired systolic function, however, benefits in women remain unclear [49, 52]. Sex-specific data for ARBs when used in ACEI-intolerant HF patients or in addition to an ACEI are limited, but candesartan and valsartan seem beneficial in women [53]. Beta-blockers carvedilol, bisoprolol, and metoprolol succinate when added to an ACEI, are beneficial in women with HF [54, 55, 56]. Aldosterone antagonists have a total mortality benefit for women with systolic HF on the basis of both the RALES (Randomized Aldactone Evaluation Study) and EPHESUS (Epleronone Post-Acute Myocardial Infarction Heart Failure Efficacy and Survival Study) trials [57, 58]. The combination of hydralazine and isosorbide dinitrates studied in the A-HeFT (African-American Heart Failure Trial) study showed significant survival benefits and fewer hospital stays for both women and men [59]. Digoxin reduces HF hospital stay with no survival benefits; levels between 0.5 and 0.9 ng/ml were considered safe for both women and men (HR: 0.8) [60, 61]. Although few studies have reported sex-specific data, it seems that cardiac resynchronization therapy (CRT) is beneficial for both women and men [62, 63]; however in women ICD do not clearly demonstrate a mortality benefit [64,65]. According to a single study women were more likely than men to require a right ventricular Assist Device (VAD) after implantation of a left VAD [66, 67]. In U.S. for 2007, women donated 28% of the available hearts and received 26% of the hearts transplanted and overall survival after transplantation on the basis of UNOS (United Network of Organ Sharing) data from 1997 to 2004 was slightly worse for women [68]. The most recent data (2007) from the International Society for Heart and Lung Transplantation showed that gender of the donor or recipient did not significantly affect 1-year mortality but that the relative ratio of 5-, 10-, and 15-year mortality was slightly higher for male recipients who received female hearts [69].

Outcomes

In terms of HF associated morbidity, women have lower quality of life than men, with more functional capacity impairment [70], more HF hospital stays [42, 43,70] and depression [71]. Men with HF have shorter survival than women [72, 73].

ATRIAL FIBRILLATION IN WOMEN

Atrial fibrillation (AF) is a supraventricular tachyarrhythmia characterized by uncoordinated atrial activation consequently reducing mechanical function leading to hemodynamic impairment, thromboembolic events contributing to significant morbidity, mortality, and cost. Gender differences exist in prevalence, symptoms and management of AF.

Epidemiology

The Global Burden of Disease Study estimated in 2010 a prevalence of AF of 373.1/100,000 for women and 596.2/100,000 for men [74]. The highest incidences and prevalence of the disease are registered in developed countries due to older mean age of the population and to better surveillance, as opposed to in developing countries where incidence and prevalence are lower [74]. Despite the higher incidence of AF in men, prevalence of the disease among women increases among elderly as a consequence of their longer lifespan [75-78]. Women are hospitalized for longer days with AF later in life than men, with greatest burden in female octogenarians and more likely to be discharged to a skilled nursing facility as compared to men [79].

EORP-AF survey (n = 3119) reported older females (≥75 years)with no difference in proportion of AF subtype (paroxysmal, persistent, permanent, etc.) in comparison to men [80].In another study conducted in Germany (n=2742) women had more frequent paroxysmal and less frequently permanent AF [81].

Risk Factors, Diagnosis and Prognosis

Women are less likely than men to have diabetes, chronic kidney disease, and obesity and more likely to have a history of stroke, heart failure, depression, and hypertension [79]. Hyperthyroidism, and prior bleeding event were not significantly different between males and females [80].Systolic BP is a better predictor of AF in women than diastolic BP [82]. HF with preserved ejection fraction (HFpEF)was more common in females [80]. Social and psychological differences between men and women contribute to AF. Women with high stress jobs are more prone to cardiovascular events [83]. Heavy alcohol consumption is associated with higher risk of AF among men, with no such association in women [84].

Coronary angiography and exercise testing was less common in females with no sex differences in transthoracic echocardiography use [80, 85].

Women suffering from AF show a different prognosis, with a higher incidence of stroke and a higher mortality rate (1.5 in men and 1.9 in women)with respect to men [86, 87, 88]. Higher mortality is mainly due to stroke and heart failure [89, 90].

Symptoms

The more common prevalent symptoms in females were palpitations and fear/anxiety. Other symptoms (e.g., dyspnoea, chest pain, fatigue, etc.) were not different between males and females. Health status scores were significantly lower for females overall, specifically for the psychological and physical domains but not for the sexual activity domain [80]. A $CHADS_2$ or CHA_2DS_2-VASc score ≥2 was more prevalent in females.Women were also more likely to experience longer symptomatic episodes, more frequent recurrences, and significantly higher ventricular rates during Afib [91].

Risk of Stroke

Women, especially those 75 years or older, have a higher risk of stroke than men, regardless of their use and adherence to warfarin [92].A higher incidence of stroke in AF women more so >75 years has been reported by several authors [93-106]. However, data from the Japanese RHYTHM Registry did not confirm the higher stroke risk in Japanese females [107]. Interestingly, women with type B blood have a 17 percent increase in stroke risk compared to men [76].

The high risk of stroke in women is contributed by-

(a) *Hypertension and Heart failure*: Although men suffer hypertension more frequently than women; the pattern changes among the elderly, and women aged >70 years typically have higher blood pressures than men [108]. A greater left ventricular wall thickness with impaired relaxation among postmenopausal women in comparison to premenopausal women has been found and confirms this association

[109].In the Framingham Heart Study, HFpEF was more frequent in women compared to men.

(b) *Hypercoagulability, Menopause andHormonal replacement therapy*: Elevated plasma levels of Von Willebrand factor and soluble E-selectin known markers of endothelial dysfunction or damage, have been associated with stroke occurrence in AF patients [110]. Von Willebrand factor levels are higher in women with respect to males [111]. Menopause doubles the risk of stroke since menopausal period is associated with severe estradiol levels and estrogen receptor reduction, increased production of inflammatory cytokines, favouring a hypercoagulable state [112]. Contradictory data are available correlating hormonal replacement treatment (HRT) and increased risk of stroke after menopause [113, 114].

(c) *Other Cardiovascular Risk Factors:* Presence of metabolic syndrome is associated with a higher stroke risk in women compared to men (30% versus 4%, respectively) [115, 116]. The sensitivity of women to alcohol damage is higher compared to men [117].

Treatment

Women tend to be more symptomatic in AF, but fare worse than men when a rhythm-control strategy is utilized with anti-arrhythmic medications.Research shows that women were prescribed beta blockers and digoxin (rate control drugs) more often, whereas men were more often prescribed class I or class III anti-arrhythmic drugs (rhythm control drugs) [118]. Procedures in women are usually recommended late as compared to men [119]. Females were less likely to have electrical cardioversion (18.9 vs. 25.5%,), and more likely to have pharmacological cardioversion (28.2 vs. 22.4%,). AF catheter ablation is successful and beneficial for selected patients of both sexes, although women may incur higher procedural bleeding complications. Women tend to be referred for AF ablation less and later than are men [79, 80, 96]. Women are over-represented in AV node ablation according to data from a small study [97].

Women have an increased risk for torsades de pointes when taking sotalol or dofetilide, and have a higher risk of bradyarrhythmias when taking antiarrhythmics.Digoxin and diuretics were more commonly used in females; with no difference in the use of beta-blockers or calcium-channel blockers [80, 120]. The amount of warfarin needed to maintain adequate anticoagulation is higher in men than in women (30 versus 25 mg per week) [121]. Lower body weight and low creatinine clearance leads to higher plasma concentration of dabigatran in females than males.Therefore, dabigatran should be used with caution in elderly women, especially if they are thin and have a reduced renal function [122, 123].

Outcomes

Females were hospitalized longer (mean days 3.6 vs 3.3), with worse Quality of life scores as compared to men, for all types of AF.Mortality for women with atrial fibrillation is up to 2.5 times greater than that for men [86].

Peripheral Arterial Disease in Women

Peripheral arterial disease (PAD) impairs quality of life and leads to high rates of morbidity and mortality. PAD is a strong marker for cardiovascular events.

Prevalence

Population studies yielded nearly equal prevalence of PAD in men and women [124]. However, there was a significant sex-based presentation for asymptomatic PAD, with a higher prevalence among women than in men (13% vs 9%; $P< .03$). PAD frequency among women may differ within elderly age groups. However, for women, the prevalence of PAD increased with age more than it did with men. In patients aged <70 years, the occurrence of PAD was 12% for women and 17% for men. Interestingly, for patients aged >85 years, women had a higher prevalence of PAD (39%) than men (27%) [125].

Risk Factors

The risk factors for PAD and CAD are comparable and include smoking, age, diabetes mellitus, hypertension and dyslipidemia [126]. Women presenting with PAD tend to be older and have dyslipidemias [127, 128]. Hypothyroidism is positively associated in men but negatively in women with

PAD [129]. Because women more often present with asymptomatic PAD and are less often diagnosed with CVD risk factors, they may not receive the same risk factor modification therapy as men [130, 131]. HRT does not appear to reduce the odds of developing PAD in postmenopausal women and may even increase the risk of morbidity from vascular interventions [132-134].

Presentation

Most studies have shown that asymptomatic severe disease is more prevalent in women than in men [127, 135, 136, 137]. McDermott et al. and others reported that about 63% of elderly women presented with no complaints of leg pain [124, 137]. Also, women presented more often with symptoms of CLI than men (13% vs 4%) with unusual signs that are ascribed to other comorbidities, such as spinal stenosis [127] accounting fewer revascularization procedures and more amputations than men. A study from the University of California found that among patients with PAD, after controlling for disease severity, women described more physical dysfunction, pain, and mood disturbances than men, leading to lower overall quality of life which may be related to depression [138,139].

Diagnosis

Most patients with PAD are asymptomatic, although use of screening questionnaires, findings of carotid or other bruits, differential blood pressure measurements, and diminished or absent peripheral pulses can help to diagnose PAD. The ankle brachial index (ABI) <0.9 is the standard screening study for the diagnosis of PAD [140]. Use of a lower ABI limit in women has been suggested to be necessary due to smaller-sized arteries in women or to the relationship between ABI and height [141]. Infact, incorporation of ABI into cardiovascular risk stratification assessment may improve the accuracy of the prediction and lead to better risk factor modification for women [142].

Treatment and Outcomes

The PAD treatment goal aims to reduce cardiovascular morbidity and mortality; improve limb-related symptoms and QoL by a combination of reduction of risk factors, medical treatment of claudication and revascularization when indicated. Smoking cessation is imperative. ACE inhibitors reduce CV risk events [143]; statins improve walking distance and in women decreased the risk of CAD and myocardial infarction and appeared to abrogate some of the detrimental effects of HRT [144].More men were receiving antiplatelet agents (58% vs.40%) and statins (87% vs.63%) than women [130, 145, 146].Men were also more likely to be selected for intervention than women [136]. Few studies indicated that women had worse 3-year graft patency results (33%) than men (49%) secondary to the fact that women had smaller infrapopliteal arteries and vein conduits than men (2.0 vs 2.5 mm) [147, 148]. HRT in postmenopausal women has been associated with worse outcomes after lower extremity revascularization [149, 150, 151, 152]. Thus women with PAD takingHRT should consider discontinuing the HRT 4 to 6 weeks before a vascular intervention [153]. Women with diabetes are at greater risk for complications than diabetic men [154, 155]. All vascular surgeries reported higher mortality and complications in women than men [156].

PREVENTION OF CARDIOVASCULAR DISEASE IN WOMEN

Substantial progress has been made in the awareness, treatment, and prevention of CVD in women since the first women-specific clinical recommendations for the prevention of CVD were published by the American Heart Associationin 1999 [1]. Approximately 50% of decline in CVD deaths has been attributed to reducing major risk factors and the other half due to secondary preventive therapies.4 Despite the gains considerable challenges remain. Table 1 presents guidelines for prevention of CVD in women [1]

Table 1. Guidelines for the prevention of CVD in women

Lifestyle Interventions
Cigarette smoking
Women should be advised not to smoke and to avoid environmental tobacco smoke. Provide counseling at each encounter, nicotine replacement, and other pharmacotherapy as indicated in conjunction with a behavioral program or formal smoking cessation program *(Class I; Level of Evidence B).*

Lifestyle Interventions
Physical activity
Women should be advised to accumulate at least 150 min/wk of moderate exercise, 75 min/wk of vigorous exercise, or an equivalent combination of moderate- and vigorous-intensity aerobic physical activity. Aerobic activity should be performed in episodes of at least 10 min, preferably spread throughout the week *(Class I; Level of Evidence B).*
Women should also be advised that additional cardiovascular benefits are provided by increasing moderate-intensity aerobic physical activity to 5 h (300 min)/wk, 2 1/2 h/wk of vigorous-intensity physical activity, or an equivalent combination of both *(Class I; Level of Evidence B).*
Women should be advised to engage in muscle-strengthening activities that involve all major muscle groups performed on ≥2 d/wk *(Class I; Level of Evidence B).*
Women who need to lose weight or sustain weight loss should be advised to accumulate a minimum of 60 to 90 min of at least moderate-intensity physical activity (e.g., brisk walking) on most, and preferably all, days of the week *(Class I; Level of Evidence B).*
Cardiac rehabilitation
A comprehensive CVD risk-reduction regimen such as cardiovascular or stroke rehabilitation or a physician-guided home- or community-based exercise training program should be recommended to women with a recent acute coronary syndrome or coronary revascularization, new-onset or chronic angina, recent cerebrovascular event, peripheral arterial disease *(Class I; Level of Evidence A)* or current/prior symptoms of heart failure and an LVEF ≤ 35% *(Class I; Level of Evidence B).*
Dietary intake
Women should be advised to consume a diet rich in fruits and vegetables; to choose whole-grain, high-fiber foods; to consume fish, especially oily fish, at least twice a week; to limit intake of saturated fat, cholesterol, alcohol, sodium, and sugar; and avoid *trans*-fatty acids. *(Class I; Level of Evidence B).*
Pregnant women should be counselled to avoid eating fish with the potential for the highest level of mercury contamination (e.g., shark, swordfish, king mackerel, or tile fish).
Weight maintenance/reduction
Women should maintain or lose weight through an appropriate balance of physical activity, caloric intake, and formal behavioural programs when indicated to maintain or achieve an appropriate body weight (BMI <25 kg/m^2 in US women), waist size (<35 in), or other target metric of obesity. *(Class I; Level of Evidence B).*
Omega-3 fatty acids
Consumption of omega-3 fatty acids in the form of fish or in capsule form (e.g., EPA 1800 mg/d) may be considered in women with hypercholesterolemia and/or hypertriglyceridemia for primary and secondary prevention *(Class IIb; Level of Evidence B).*
Major risk factor interventions
Blood pressure: optimal level and lifestyle
An optimal blood pressure of <120/80 mm Hg should be encouraged through lifestyle approaches such as weight control, increased physical activity, alcohol moderation, sodium restriction, and increased consumption of fruits, vegetables, and low-fat dairy products *(Class I; Level of Evidence B).*

Table 1. (Continued)

Major risk factor interventions
Blood pressure: pharmacotherapy
Pharmacotherapy is indicated when blood pressure is ≥140/90 mm Hg (≥130/80 mm Hg in the setting of chronic kidney disease and diabetes mellitus). Thiazide diuretics should be part of the drug regimen for most patients unless contraindicated or if there are compelling indications for other agents in specific vascular diseases. Initial treatment of high-risk women with acute coronary syndrome or MI should be with β-blockers and/or ACE inhibitors/ARBs, with addition of other drugs such as thiazides as needed to achieve goal blood pressure *(Class I; Level of Evidence A).*
Note: ACE inhibitors are contraindicated in pregnancy and ought to be used with caution in women who may become pregnant.
Lipid and lipoprotein levels: optimal levels and lifestyle
The following levels of lipids and lipoproteins in women should be encouraged through lifestyle approaches: LDL-C <100 mg/dL, HDL-C >50 mg/dL, triglycerides <150 mg/dL, and non–HDL-C (total cholesterol minus HDL) <130 mg/dL *(Class I; Level of Evidence B).*
Lipids: pharmacotherapy for LDL-C lowering, high-risk women
LDL-Clowering drug therapy is recommended simultaneously with lifestyle therapy in women with CHD to achieve LDL-C <100 mg/dL *(Class I; Level of Evidence A)* and is also indicated in women with other atherosclerotic CVD or diabetes mellitus or 10-year absolute risk >20% *(Class I; Level of Evidence B).*
A reduction to<70 mg/dL is reasonable in very-high-risk women (those with recent ACS or multiple poorly controlled cardiovascular risk factors) with CHD and may require an LDL-lowering drug combination *(Class IIa; Level of Evidence B).*
Lipids: pharmacotherapy for LDL-C lowering, other at-risk women
LDL-C–lowering with lifestyle therapy is useful if LDL-C level is ≥130 mg/dL, there are multiple risk factors, and the 10-y absolute CHD risk is 10% to 20% *(Class I; Level of Evidence B).*
LDL-C lowering is useful with lifestyle therapy if LDL-C level is ≥160 mg/dL and multiple risk factors even if 10-y absolute CHD risk is<10% *(Class I; Level of Evidence B).*
LDL-C lowering with lifestyle therapy is useful if LDL ≥190 mg/dL regardless of the presence or absence of other risk factors or CVD *(Class I; Level of Evidence B).*
In women >60 y of age and with an estimated CHD risk >10%, statins could be considered if hsCRP is >2 mg/dL after lifestyle modification and no acute inflammatory process is present *(Class IIb; Level of Evidence B).*
Lipids: pharmacotherapy for low HDL-C or elevated non–HDL-C
Niacin or fibrate therapy can be useful when HDL-C is low (<50 mg/dL) or non–HDL-C is elevated (>130 mg/dL) in high-risk women after LDL-C goal is reached *(Class IIb; Level of Evidence B).*
Diabetes mellitus
Lifestyle and pharmacotherapy can be useful in women with diabetes mellitus to achieve an HbA_{1C} <7% if this can be accomplished without significant hypoglycemia *(Class IIa; Level of Evidence B).*

Preventive drug interventions
Aspirin: high-risk women
Aspirin therapy (75–325 mg/d) should be used in women with CHD unless contraindicated *(Class I; Level of Evidence A).*
Aspirin therapy (75–325 mg/d) is reasonable in women with diabetes mellitus unless contraindicated *(Class IIa; Level of Evidence B).*
If a high-risk woman has an indication but is intolerant of aspirin therapy, clopidogrel should be substituted *(Class I; Level of Evidence B).*
Aspirin: other at-risk or healthy women
Aspirin therapy can be useful in women ≥65 y of age (81 mg daily or 100 mg every other day) if blood pressure is controlled and benefit for ischemic stroke and MI prevention is likely to outweigh risk of gastrointestinal bleeding and hemorrhagic stroke *(Class IIa; Level of Evidence B)* and may be reasonable for women <65 y of age for ischemic stroke prevention *(Class IIb; Level of Evidence B).*
Aspirin: atrial fibrillation
Aspirin 75–325 mg should be used in women with chronic or paroxysmal atrial fibrillation with a contraindication to warfarin or at low risk of stroke (<1%/y or CHADS2 score of <2) *(Class I; Level of Evidence A).*
Warfarin: atrial fibrillation
For women with chronic or paroxysmal atrial fibrillation, warfarin should be used to maintain the INR at 2.0 to 3.0 unless they are considered to be at low risk for stroke (<1%/y or high risk of bleeding) *(Class I; Level of Evidence A).*
Dabigatran: atrial fibrillation
Dabigatran is useful as an alternative to warfarin for the prevention of stroke and systemic thromboembolism in patients with paroxysmal to permanent AF and risk factors for stroke or systemic embolization who do not have a prosthetic heart valve or hemodynamically significant valve disease, severe renal failure (creatinineclearance < 15 mL/min), or advanced liver disease (impaired baseline clotting function) *(Class I; Level of Evidence B).*
β-Blockers
β-Blockers should be used for up to 12 mo *(Class I; Level of Evidence A)* or up to 3 y *(Class I; Level of Evidence B)* in all women after MI or ACS with normal left ventricular function unless contraindicated.
Long-term β-blocker therapy should be used indefinitely for women with left ventricular failure unless contraindications are present *(Class I; Level of Evidence A).*
Long-term β-blocker therapy may be considered in other women with coronary or vascular disease and normal left ventricular function *(Class IIb; Level of Evidence C).*
ACE inhibitors/ARBs
ACE inhibitors should be used (unless contraindicated) in women after MI and in those with clinical evidence of heart failure, LVEF ≤ 40%, or diabetes mellitus *(Class I; Level of Evidence A).*

Table 1. (Continued)

Preventive drug interventions
In women after MI and in those with clinical evidence of heart failure, an LVEF ≤ 40%, or diabetes mellitus who are intolerant of ACE inhibitors, ARBs should be used instead *(Class I; Level of Evidence B).*
Note: ACE inhibitors are contraindicated in pregnancy and ought to be used with caution in women who may become pregnant.
Aldosterone blockade
Use of aldosterone blockade (e.g., spirololactone) after MI is indicated in women who do not have significant hypotension, renal dysfunction, or hyperkalemia who are already receiving therapeutic doses of an ACE inhibitor and β-blocker and have LVEF ≤ 40% with symptomatic heart failure *(Class I; Level of Evidence B).*

Conclusion

CVD remains a leading cause of mortality in women. Considerable progress has been achieved with women specific guidelines and participation of women in clinical trials.A better understanding of biological differences affecting pathological manifestations influencing prevention and treatment plans need to be tailor made to improve CVD health care in women. Guidelines to specific areas of CVD like heart failure, atrial fibrillation, valvular and structural disease, peripheral vascular disease and cerebro-vascular should be laid considering existing gender differences.

References

[1] Lori Mosca, Emelia, JB; Kathy, BJ; Bezanson, RJ; Dolor, DM; Lloyd-Jones, Newby, LK; et al., Effectiveness-Based Guidelines for the Prevention of Cardiovascular Disease in Women—2011 Update A Guideline From the *American Heart Association Circulation*, Mar 22, 2011, 123(11), 1243-1262.

[2] Pepine, CJ; Kerensky, RA; Lambert, CR; Smith, KM; von Mering, GO; Sopko, G; et al. "Some thoughts on the Vasculopathy of Women with Ischemic Heart Disease". *J Am CollCardiol.*, 2006, 47(suppl), S30-S35.

[3] Shaw, LJ; Bugiardini, R; Bairey Merz, CN. "Women and Ischemic Heart Disease". *J Am CollCardiol*, 2009, 54,1561-75.

[4] Jacobs, AK. Coronary intervention, "Are Women No Different than Men?" *Circ Cardiovascular Intervent*, 2009, 2,69-78.

[5] Huxley, VH. "Sex and the Cardiovascular System: The Intriguing Tale of How Women and Men Regulate Cardiovascular Function Differently". *Adv Physiol Educ*, 2007, 31,17-22.

[6] Lang, TJ. Estrogen as an immunomodulator. *Clin Immunol.*, 2004 Dec,113(3),224-30.

[7] Mendelsohn, ME; Karas, RH. The protective effects of estrogen on the cardiovascular system. *N Engl J Med.*, 1999, 340, 1801–1811.

[8] Lansky, AJ; Hochman, JS; Ward, PA; Minzgs, Fabunmi, R; Berger, PB; etal., "Percutaneous Coronary Interventio and Adjunctive Pharmacotherapy in Women", *A statement for healthcare professionals from the American Heart Association Circulation*, 2005, 111,940-53.

[9] Akutsu, PD; Snowden, LR; Organista, KC. Referral patterns to ethnic-specific and mainstream mental health programs for Hispanics and non-Hispanic Whites *Journal of Counseling Psychology*, 1996, 43(1),4356–64.

[10] Samad, A; Wang, TY; Fraizer, CG; Shah, SH; Dolor, RJ; Newby, LK. "Closing the Gap: Treating Hypertension in Women", *Cardiol Rev*, 2008, 16(6),305-13.

[11] Goldschmid, MG; Barrett-Connor, E; Edelstein, SL; et al. Dyslipidemia and ischemic heart disease mortality among men and women with diabetes. *Circulation*, 1994, 89(3),991-997.

[12] Seeman, T; Mendes de Leon, C; Berkman, L; Ostfeld, A. Risk factors for coronary heart disease among older men and women: a prospective study of community-dwelling elderly. *Am J Epidemiol*, 1993, 138,1037-1049.

[13] Barrett Connor, EL; Cohn, BA; Wingard, DL; Edelstein, SL. Why is diabetes mellitus a stronger risk factor for fatal ischemic heart disease in women than in men? The Rancho Bernardo Study. *J Am Med Assoc*, 1991, 265,627-631.

[14] Donahue, RP; Goldberg, RJ; Chen, Z; Gore, JM; Alpert, JS. Theinfluence of sex and diabetes mellitus on survival following acute myocardial infarction: a community-wide perspective. *J ClinEpidemiol*, 1993, 46,245-252.

[15] Sowers, JR. "Diabetes mellitus and cardiovascular disease in women", *Arch Intern Med*, 1998 Mar 23, 158(6),617-621.

[16] Garcia, MJ; Namara, Mc; Gordon, PM; TKannel, WB. "Morbidity and mortality in diabetics in the Framingham population: sixteen-year follow-up study", *Diabetes Care.*, 1990, 13,631- 654.

[17] Capron, L; Jarnet, J; Kusandjian, S; Honsait, E. Growth promoting effects of diabetes and insulin on arteries. *Diabetes*, 1986 Sep, 35(90),973- 978.

[18] Oppenheimer, MJ; Sundquist, K; Bierman, EL. "Down-regulation of high-density lipoprotein receptor in human fibroblasts by insulin and IGF-1", *Diabetes*, 1989 Jan, 38(1),117- 122.

[19] Kuhn, FE; Rackley, CE. Coronary artery disease in women. Risk factors, evaluation, treatment, and prevention. *Arch Intern Med*, 1993 Dec, 153(23),2626-2636.

[20] Tremollieres, FA; Pouilles, JM; Cauneille, C; Ribot, C. Coronary heart disease risk factors and menopause: a study in 1684 French women. *Atherosclerosis*, 1999, 142,415-423.

[21] Brown, SA; Hutchinson, R; Morrisett, J; et al. Plasma lipid, lipoprotein cholesterol, and a poprotein distributions in selected US communities. The Atherosclerosis Risk in Communities (ARIC) Study, *Arterioscler Thromb*, 1993, 13,1139-1158.

[22] Davis, CE; Pajak, A; Rywik, S. etal. Natural menopause and cardiovascular disease risk factors. The Poland and US Collaborative Study on Cardiovascular Disease Epidemiology. *Ann Epidemiol*, 1994, 4,445-448.

[23] Michael, Miller; Neil, J; Stone, Christie; Ballantyne, Vera; Bittner, Michael, H; Criqui, Henry, N; Ginsberg, Anne, Carol; Goldberg, William; James, Howard; Marc, S. Jacobson, Penny, M. Kris-Etherton, Terry, A. Lennie, Moshe Levi, Theodore Mazzone, Subramanian Pennathur; Triglycerides and Cardiovascular Disease, *Circulation.*, 2011,123,2292-2333.

[24] Hokanson, JE; Austin, MA. Plasma triglyceride level is a risk factor for cardiovascular disease independent of high-density lipoprotein cholesterol level: a meta-analysis of population-based prospective studies. *J Cardiovasc Risk*, 1996, 3(2),213-9.

[25] Expert Panel on Detection, Evaluation, and Treatment of High Blood Cholesterol in Adults (Adult Treatment Panel III). Third Report of the National Cholesterol Education Program (NCEP) Expert Panel on Detection, Evaluation, and Treatment of High Blood Cholesterol in Adults (Adult Treatment Panel III) final report. *Circulation*, 2002, 106,3143-3421.

[26] Weissman, MM; Bland, R; Joyce, PR; Newman, S; Wells, JE; Wittchen, HU. "Sex Differences in Rates of Depression: Cross-National Perspectives" *J Affect Disord.*, 1993 October-November, 29(2-3),77-84.

[27] Kessler, RC; McGonagle, KA; Swartz, M.; Blazer, DG; Nelson, CB. "Sex and Depression in the National Comorbidity Survey. I: Lifetime Prevalence, Chronicity and Recurrence," *J Affect Disord.*,1993,2-3, 85–96.

[28] Parloop, Bhatt; Aditi, Patel; Parth, Parikh; Jawahar, Mehta; Piyush, Thakar; Aditi, Nanavati; Roosha, Parikh; Apurva, Patel; Keyur, Parikh; Depression and Outcome of Patients with Acute Coronary Syndrome: A 3 Year Follow-up Study, *JACC*, 2015 March 17, Volume 65, Issue 10S, A1383.

[29] Lorna, E; Clarson, Samantha, L; Hider, John; Belcher; Carl, Heneghan; Edward, Roddy; Christian, D. Mallen, Increased risk of vascular disease associated with gout: a retrospective, matched cohort study in the UK Clinical Practice Research Datalink, *Ann Rheum Dis*, 2015, 74,642-647.

[30] Hermes, W; Van Kesteren, F; De Groot, CJ, "Preeclampsia and Cardiovascular Risk," *Minerva Ginecol*, 2012 August, 64(4),281-92.

[31] Bellamy, L; et al., "Pre-Eclampsia and Risk of CVD and Cancer in Later Life: Systematic Review and Meta-Analysis," *BMJ*, 2007, 335(7627), p. 974.

[32] Mokdad, AH; Ford, ES; Bowman, BA. Prevalence of obesity, diabetes, and obesity-related health risk factors, 2001. *JAMA.*, 2003 Jan 1, 289,76-79.

[33] Haffner, SM; Lehto, S; Ronnemaa, T; Pyorala, K; Laakso, M. "Mortality from Coronary Heart Disease in Subjects with Type 2 Diabetes and in Nondiabetic Subjects with and without Prior Myocardial Infarction," *N Engl J Med*, 1998, 339, 229-234.

[34] Coustan, DR; Carpenter, MW; O'Sullivan, PS; Carr, SR; "Gestational Diabetes: Predictors of Subsequent Disordered Glucose Metabolism", *Am J Obstet Gynecol*, 1993, 168, 1139-1144.

[35] Kjos, SL; Peters, RK; Xiang, A; Henry, OA; Montoro, M; Buchanan, TA. "Predicting Future Diabetes in Latino Women with Gestational Diabetes. Utility of Early Postpartum Glucose Tolerance Testing," *Diabetes*, 1995, 44, 586-591.

[36] Sullivan, SD; Umans, JG; Ratner, R. Gestational diabetes: Implications for cardiovascular health. *Curr Diab Rep.*, 2012, 12(1),43–52.

[37] Tarim, E; Yigit, F; Kilicdag, E; Bagis, T; Demircan, S; Simsek, E; Haydardedeoglu, B; Yanik, F. Early onset of subclinical atherosclerosis

in women with gestational diabetes mellitus. *Ultrasound Obstet Gynecol.*, 2006, 27(2),177–182.

[38] Victor Guetta; Richard, O. Cannon, Cardiovascular Effects of Estrogen and Lipid-Lowering Therapies in Postmenopausal Women, *Circulation.*, 1996, 93,1928-1937.

[39] Lori, Mosca; Peter, Collins; David, M; Herrington, Michael, E. Mendelsohn, Richard, C; Pasternak, Rose; Marie, Robertson; Karin, Schenck-Gustafsson; Sidney, C; Smith, Kathryn, A; Taubert, Nanette, K. Wenger, Hormone Replacement Therapy and Cardiovascular Disease; *Circulation*, July 24, 2001, 499-503.

[40] Beral, V; Banks, E; Reeves, G. Appleby PUse of HRT and the subsequent risk of cancer. *Journal of Epidemiology and Biostatistics*, 1999, 4(3),191-210, 210-5

[41] Irwin Klein, Sara Danzi, Thyroid hormone treatment to mend a broken heart, *J clin Endocrino Metabo*, 2008, 93(4), 1172-1174.

[42] Eileen, MH; Ileana, LP. *Heart failure in women JACC*, 2009, 54(6), 491-498.

[43] Galvao, M; Kalman, J; DeMarco, T. Gender differences in in-hospital management and outcomes in patients with decompensated heart failure: analysis from the Acute Decompensated Heart Failure National Registry (ADHERE). *J Card Fail.*, 2006 Mar, 12(2),100-107.

[44] Redfield, MM; Jacobsen, SJ; Burnett, JC; Jr. Mahoney, DW; Bailey, KR; Rodeheffer, RJ. Burden of systolic and diastolic ventricular dysfunction in the community: appreciating the scope of the heart failure epidemic. *JAMA.*, 2003 Jan 8, 289(2),194-202.

[45] Vasan, RS; Larson, MG; Benjamin, EJ; Evans, JC; Reiss, CK; Levy, D. Congestive heart failure in subjects with normal versus reduced left ventricular ejection fraction: prevalence and mortality in a population-based cohort. *J Am Coll Cardiol.*, 1999 June,33(7),1948-1955.

[46] Nieminen, MS; Harjola, VP; Hochadel, M. Gender related differences in patients presenting with acute heart failure. Results from EuroHeart Failure Survey II *Eur J Heart Fail.*, 2008 Feb, 10(2),140-148.

[47] O''Meara, E; Clayton, T; McEntegart, MB. Sex differences in clinical characteristics and prognosis in a broad spectrum of patients with heart failure: results of the Candesartan in Heart failure: Assessment of Reduction in Mortality and morbidity (CHARM) program. *Circulation.*, 2007 Jan 19, 115(24),3111-3120.

[48] Ntusi, NB; Mayosi, BM. Aetiology and risk factors of peripartum cardiomyopathy: a systematic review. *Int J Cardiol.*, 2009 Jan 9, 131(2),168-179.
[49] Hunt, SA; Abraham, WT; Chin, MH. 2009 focused update incorporated into the ACC/AHA 2005 guidelines for the diagnosis and management of heart failure in adults: a report of the American College of Cardiology Foundation/American Heart Association Task Force on Practice Guidelines. *J Am CollCardiol.*, 2009, 53(15),e1-e90.
[50] Johnstone, D; Limacher, M; Rousseau, M. Clinical characteristics of patients in studies of left ventricular dysfunction (SOLVD). *Am J Cardiol.*,1992 Oct 1, 70(9),894-900.
[51] Wang, TJ; Larson, MG; Levy, D. Impact of age and sex on plasma natriuretic peptide levels in healthy adults. *Am J Cardiol.*, 2002 Aug 1, 90(3),254-258.
[52] The CONSENSUS Trial Study Group. Effects of enalapril on mortality in severe congestive heart failure. Results of the Cooperative North Scandinavian Enalapril Survival Study (CONSENSUS). *N Engl J Med.*, 1987, 316,1429-1435.
[53] Young, JB; Dunlap, ME; Pfeffer, MA. Mortality and morbidity reduction with Candesartan in patients with chronic heart failure and left ventricular systolic dysfunction: results of the CHARM low-left ventricular ejection fraction trials. *Circulation.*, 2004, 110,2618-2626.
[54] Packer, M; Bristow, MR; Cohn, JN; Carvedilol, US. Heart Failure Study Group The effect of carvedilol on morbidity and mortality in patients with chronic heart failure. *N Engl J Med.*, 1996, 334,1349-1355.
[55] Packer, M; Coats, AJ; Fowler, MB. Effect of carvedilol on survival in severe chronic heart failure. *N Engl J Med.*, 2001, 344,1651-1658.
[56] Ghali, JK; Pina ,IL; Gottlieb, SS; Deedwania, PC; Wikstrand, JC. Metoprolol CR/XL in female patients with heart failure: analysis of the experience in Metoprolol Extended-Release Randomized Intervention Trial in Heart Failure (MERIT-HF). *Circulation.*,2002, 105,1585-1591.
[57] Pitt, B; Zannad, F; Remme, WJ. Randomized Aldactone Evaluation Study Investigators The effect of spironolactone on morbidity and mortality in patients with severe heart failure. *N Engl J Med.*, 1999, 341,709-717.
[58] Pitt, B; Remme, W; Zannad, F. Eplerenone, a selective aldosterone blocker, in patients with left ventricular dysfunction after myocardial infarction. *N Engl J Med.*, 2003, 348,1309-1321.

[59] Taylor, AL; Lindenfeld, J; Ziesche, S. Outcomes by gender in the African-American Heart Failure Trial. *J Am Coll Cardiol.*, 2006, 48,2263-2267.

[60] The Digitalis Investigation Group. The effect of digoxin on mortalitymorbidity in patients with heart failure. *N Engl J Med.*, 1997, 336,525-533.

[61] Adams, KF; Jr. Patterson, JH; Gattis, WA. Relationship of serum digoxin concentration to mortality and morbidity in women in the digitalis investigation group trial: a retrospective analysis. *J Am Coll Cardiol.*, 2005 Aug 2, 46(3),497-504.

[62] Bristow, MR; Saxon, LA; Boehmer, J. Cardiac-resynchronization therapy with or without an implantable defibrillator in advanced chronic heart failure. *N Engl J Med.*, 2004, 350,2140-2150.

[63] Cleland, JG; Daubert, JC; Erdmann, E. The effect of cardiac resynchronization on morbidity and mortality in heart failure. *N Engl J Med.*, 2005, 352,1539-1549.

[64] Bardy, GH; Lee, KL; Mark, DB. Amiodarone or an implantable cardioverter-defibrillator for congestive heart failure. *N Engl J Med.*, 2005, 352,225-237.

[65] Zareba, W; Moss, AJ; Jackson Hall, W. Clinical course and implantable cardioverter defibrillator therapy in postinfarction women with severe left ventricular dysfunction. *J Cardiovasc Electrophysiol.*, 2005, 16,1265-1270.

[66] Ochiai, Y; McCarthy, PM; Smedira, NG. Predictors of severe right ventricular failure after implantable left ventricular assist device insertion: analysis of 245 patients. *Circulation.*, 2002, 106,I198-I202.

[67] Morgan, JA; Weinberg, AD; Hollingsworth, KW; Flannery, MR; Oz, MC; Naka, Y. Effect of gender on bridging to transplantation and posttransplantation survival in patients with left ventricular assist devices. *J Thorac Cardiovasc Surg.*, 2004, 127,1193-1195.

[68] Organ Procurement and Transplantation Network. http:// optn.transplant. hrsa.gov/l atestData/step2.asp. Accessed Jan 16; 2016.

[69] International Society for Heart and Lung Transplantation. http:// www. ishlt.org/registries/slides.asp?slides=heartLungRegistry. *Accessed Jan*, 16 2016.

[70] Deswal, A; Bozkurt, B. Comparison of morbidity in women versus men with heart failure and preserved ejection fraction. *Am J Cardiol.*, 2006, 97,1228-1231.

[71] Gottlieb, SS; Khatta, M; Friedmann, E. The influence of age, gender, and race on the prevalence of depression in heart failure patients. *J Am Coll Cardiol.*, 2004, 43,1542-1549.

[72] Roger, VL; Weston, SA; Redfield, MM. Trends in heart failure incidence and survival in a community-based population. *JAMA.*, 2004, 292,344-350.

[73] Levy, D; Kenchaiah, S; Larson, MG. Long-term trends in the incidence of and survival with heart failure. *N Engl J Med.*, 2002, 347,1397-1402.

[74] Chugh, SS; Havmoeller, R; Narayanan, K; et al. Worldwide epidemiology of atrial fibrillation: a Global Burden of Disease 2010 Study. *Circulation.*, 2014, 129(8),837–847.

[75] European Heart Rhythm Association, European Association for Cardio-Thoracic Surgery, Camm AJ. Guidelines for the management of atrial fibrillation: the Task Force for the Management of Atrial Fibrillation of the European Society of Cardiology (ESC). *Eur Heart J.*, 2010 Oct, 31(19),2369–2429.

[76] Qi, L; et al. ABO Blood Group and Risk of Stroke in US Men and Women. Abstract 16887. *American Heart Association*, 16 Nov. 2011.

[77] Mason, PK; Moorman, L; Lake, D; et al. Gender and racial characteristics of patients referred to a tertiary atrial fibrillation center. *JAFIB.*, 2010, 2(3),827.

[78] Daniela Poli and Emilia Antonucci. Epidemiology, diagnosis, and management of atrial fibrillation in women, *Int J Womens Health.*, 2015 Jun 11,7, 605–614.

[79] Zoni-Berisso, M; Lercari, F; Carazza, T; Domenicucci, S. Epidemiology of atrial fibrillation: European perspective. *Clin Epidemiol.*, 2014, 6,213–220.

[80] Daniela Poli, Emilia Antonucci, Epidemiology, diagnosis, and management of atrial fibrillation in women,*International Journal of Women's Health*, 2015,7 605–614.

[81] Bosch, RF; Pittrow, D; Beltzer, A; Kruck, I; Kirch, W; Kohlhaussen, A; Bonnemeier, H. Gender differences in patients with atrial fibrillation. *Herzschrittmacherther Elektrophysiol.*, 2013 Sep, 24(3),176-83.

[82] Sullivan, RM; Zhang, J; Zamba, G; Lip, GY; Olshansky, B. Relation of gender-specific risk of ischemic stroke in patients with atrial fibrillation to differences in warfarin anticoagulation control (from AFFIRM). *Am J Cardiol*, 2012, 110,1799-802.

[83] Slopen, N; Glynn, RJ; Buring, JE; Lewis, TT; Williams, DR; Albert, MA. Job strain, job insecurity, and incident cardiovascular disease in the

women's health study: results from a 10-year prospective study. *PLoS One*., 2012, 7(7),40-512.

[84] Mukamal, KJ; Tolstrup, JS; Friberg, J; Jensen, G; Grønbaek, M. Alcohol consumption and risk of atrial fibrillation in men and women: the Copenhagen City Heart Study. *Circulation*., 2005, 112(12),1736-1742.

[85] Stöllberger, C; Chnupa, P; Kronik, G; et al. Transesophageal echocardiography to assess embolic risk in patients with atrial fibrillation. ELAT Study Group. Embolism in Left Atrial Thrombi. *Ann Intern Med*., 1998, 128(8),630–638.

[86] Michelena, HI; Powell, BD; Brady, PA; Friedman, PA; Ezekowitz, MD. Gender in atrial fibrillation: ten years later. *Gend Med*., 2010, 3(7),206-217.

[87] Benjamin, EJ; Wolf, PA; D'Agostino, RB; Silbershatz, H; Kannel, WB; Levy, D. Impact of atrial fibrillation on the risk of death: the Framingham Heart Study. *Circulation*., 1998, 98(10),946–952.

[88] Wagstaff, AJ; Overard, TF; Lip, GY; Lane, DA. Is female sex a risk factor for stroke and thromboembolism in patients with atrial fibrillation? A systematic review and meta-analysis. *QJM*., 2014, 107 (12),955–967.

[89] Swedberg, K; Cleland, J; Dargie, H; et al. Guidelines for the diagnosis and treatment of chronic heart failure: executive summary (update 2005): The Task Force for the Diagnosis and Treatment of Chronic Heart Failure of the European Society of Cardiology. *Eur Heart J*., 2005, 26(11),1115–1140.

[90] Pisters, R; Lane, DA; Marin, F; Camm, AJ; Lip, GY. Stroke and thromboembolism in atrial fibrillation. *Circ J*, 2012, 76,2289-304.

[91] Roy, D; Talajic, M; Dorian, P; et al. Amiodarone to prevent recurrence of atrial fibrillation. Canadian Trial of Atrial Fibrillation Investigators. *N Engl J Med*., 2000, 342(13),913-920.

[92] Avgil Tsadok, M; Jackevicius, CA; Rahme, E; Humphries, KH; Behlouli, H; Pilote, L. Sex differences in stroke risk among older patients with recently diagnosed atrial fibrillation. *JAMA*., 2012, 307(18),1952-1195.

[93] Fang, MC; Singer, DE; Chang, Y; et al. Gender differences in the risk of ischemic stroke and peripheral embolism in atrial fibrillation: the AnTicoagulation and Risk factors In Atrial fibrillation (ATRIA) study. *Circulation*., 2005, 112,1687-1691.

[94] Sullivan, RM; Zhang, J; Zamba, G; Lip, GY; Olshansky, B. Relation of gender-specific risk of ischemic stroke in patients with atrial fibrillation

to differences in warfarin anticoagulation control (from AFFIRM). *Am J Cardiol.*, 2012, 110(12),1799-1802.

[95] Madias, C; Trohman, RG. The link between atrial fibrillation and stroke in women. *Womens Health (LondEngl).*, 2011, 7(3),375–382.

[96] Dagres, N; Nieuwlaat, R; Vardas, PE; et al. Gender-related differences in presentation, treatment, and outcome of patients with atrial fibrillation in Europe: a report from the Euro Heart Survey on Atrial Fibrillation. *J Am Coll Cardiol.*, 2007, 49,572-577.

[97] Forleo, GB; Tondo, C; De Luca, L; et al. Gender-related differences in catheter ablation of atrial fibrillation. *Europace.*, 2007, 9(8),613–620.

[98] Mant, J; Hobbs, FD; Fletcher, K; et al. Warfarin versus aspirin for stroke prevention in an elderly community population with atrial fibrillation (the Birmingham Atrial Fibrillation Treatment of the Aged Study, BAFTA): a randomised controlled trial. *Lancet.*, 2007, 370(9586),493–503.

[99] Dagres, N; Nieuwlaat, R; Vardas, PE; et al. Gender-related differences in presentation, treatment, and outcome of patients with atrial fibrillation in Europe: a report from the Euro Heart Survey on Atrial Fibrillation. *J Am Coll Cardiol.*, 2007, 49(5),572–577.

[100] Poli, D; Antonucci, E; Grifoni, E; Abbate, R; Gensini, GF; Prisco, D. Gender differences in stroke risk of atrial fibrillation patients on oral anticoagulant treatment. *ThrombHaemost.*, 2009, 101(5),938–942.

[101] Lip, GY; Frison, L; Halperin, JL; Lane, DA. Identifying patients at high risk for stroke despite anticoagulation: a comparison of contemporary stroke risk stratification schemes in an anticoagulated atrial fibrillation cohort. *Stroke.*, 2010, 41(12),2731–2738.

[102] Van Staa, TP; Setakis, E; Di Tanna, GL; Lane, DA; Lip, GY. A comparison of risk stratification schemes for stroke in 79, 884 atrial fibrillation patients in general practice. *J Thromb Haemost.*, 2011, 9(1),39–48.

[103] Olesen, JB; Lip, GY; Hansen, ML; et al. Validation of risk stratification schemes for predicting stroke and thromboembolism in patients with atrial fibrillation: nationwide cohort study. *BMJ.*, 2011 Jan 31, 342,d124.

[104] Mikkelsen, AP; Lindhardsen, J; Lip, GY; Gislason, GH; Torp-Pedersen, C; Olesen, JB. Female sex as a risk factor for stroke in atrial fibrillation: a nationwide cohort study. *J Thromb Haemost.*, 2012, 10(9),1745–1751.

[105] Avgil Tsadok, M; Jackevicius, CA; Rahme, E; Humphries, KH; Behloulim H; Pilote, L. Sex differences in stroke risk among older

patients with recently diagnosed atrial fibrillation. *JAMA.*, 2012, 307(18),1952–1958.

[106] Friberg, L; Benson, L; Rosenqvist, M; Lip, GY. Assessment of female sex as a risk factor in atrial fibrillation in Sweden, nationwide retrospective cohort study. *BMJ.*, 2012, 344,e3522.

[107] JCS, Joint Working Group. Guidelines for Pharmacotherapy of Atrial Fibrillation (JCS 2013). *Circ J.*, 2014, 78(8),1997–2021.

[108] Franklin, S; Gustin, W; 4th, Wong, ND; et al. Haemodynamic patterns of age-related changes in blood pressure. The Framingham Heart Study. *Circulation.*, 1997, 96(1),308–315.

[109] Hinderliter, A; Sherwood, A; Blumenthal, JA; et al. Changes in hemodynamics and left ventricular structure after menopause. *Am J Cardiol.*, 2002, 89(7),830–833.

[110] Krishnamoorthy, S; Khoo, CW; Lim, HS; et al. Prognostic role of plasma von Willebrand factor and soluble E-selectin levels for future cardiovascular events in a 'real-world' community cohort of patients with atrial fibrillation. *Eur J Clin Invest.*, 2013, 43(10),1032–1038.

[111] Conway, DS; Heeringa, J; Van Der Kuip, DA; et al. Atrial fibrillation and the prothrombotic state in the elderly: the Rotterdam Study. *Stroke.*, 2003, 34(2),413–417.

[112] Cove, CL; Albert, CM; Andreotti, F; Badimon, L; Van Gelder, IC; Hylek, EM. Female sex as an independent risk factor for stroke in atrial fibrillation: possible mechanisms. *Thromb Haemost.*, 2014, 111(3), 385–391.

[113] Magliano, DJ; Rogers, SL; Abramson, MJ; Tonkin, AM. Hormone therapy and cardiovascular disease: a systematic review and meta-analysis. *BJOG.*, 2006, 113(1),5–14.

[114] Viscoli, CM; Brass, LM; Kernan, WN; Sarrel, PM; Suissa, S; Horwitz, RI. A clinical trial of estrogen-replacement therapy after ischemic stroke. *N Engl J Med.*, 2001, 345(17),1243–1249.

[115] Najarian, RM; Sullivan, LM; Kannel, WB; Wilson, PW; D'Agostino, RB; Wolf, PA. Metabolic syndrome compared with type 2 diabetes mellitus as a risk factor for stroke: the Framingham Offspring Study. *Arch Intern Med.*, 2006, 166(1),106–111.

[116] Boden-Albala, B; Sacco, RL; Lee, HS; et al. Metabolic syndrome and ischemic stroke risk: Northern Manhattan Study. *Stroke.*, 2008, 39(1),30–35.

[117] White, IR; Altmann, DR; Nanchahal, K. Alcohol consumption and mortality: modelling risks for men and women at different ages. *BMJ.*, 2002, 325(7357),191.

[118] Oza, NM; Baveja, S; Tedrow, U. Bridging the gender gap in atrial fibrillation. *Expert Rev Cardiovasc Ther.*, 2015, 13(3),317–323.

[119] Volgman, AS; Manankil, MF; Mookherjee, D; Trohman, RG. Women with atrial fibrillation, greater risk, less attention. *Gend Med.*, 2009, 6(3),419-32.

[120] Michelena, HI; Powell, BD; Brady, PA; Friedman, PA; Ezekowitz, MD. Gender in atrial fibrillation: Ten years later. *Med. Gend Med.*, 2010 Jun, 7(3),206-17.

[121] Garcia, D; Regan, S; Crowther, M; Hughes, RA; Hylek, EM. Warfarin maintenance dosing patterns in clinical practice: implications for safer anticoagulation in the elderly population. *Chest.*, 2005, 127(6),2049–2056.

[122] Reilly, PA; Lehr, T; Haertter, S; et al. The effect of dabigatran plasma concentrations and patient characteristics on the frequency of ischemic stroke and major bleeding in atrial fibrillation patients: the RE-LY Trial (Randomized Evaluation of Long-Term Anticoagulation Therapy). *J Am Coll Cardiol.*, 2014, 63(4),321–328.

[123] Pengo, V; Crippa, L; Falanga, A; et al. Questions and answers on the use of dabigatran and perspectives on the use of other new oral anti-coagulants in patients with atrial fibrillation. A consensus document of the Italian Federation of Thrombosis Centers (FCSA). *Thromb Haemost.*, 2011, 106(5),868–876.

[124] Sigvant, B; Wiberg-Hedman, K; Bergqvist, D; Rolandsson, O; Andersson, B; Persson, E; et al. A population-based study of peripheral arterial disease prevalence with special focus on critical limb ischemia and sex differences. *J Vasc Surg*, 2007, 45,1185-91.

[125] Diehm, C; Schuster, A; Allenberg, JR; Darius, H; Haberl, R; Lange, S; et al. High prevalence of peripheral arterial disease and co-morbidity in 6880 primary care patients: cross-sectional study. *Atherosclerosis*, 2004, 172,95-105.

[126] Lloyd-Jones, D; Adams, R; Carnethon, M; De, SG; Ferguson, TB; Flegal, K; et al. Heart disease and stroke statistics–2009 update: a report from the American Heart Association Statistics Committee and Stroke Statistics Subcommittee. *Circulation*, 2009, 119,e21-181.

[127] Brevetti, G; Bucur, R; Balbarini, A; Melillo, E; Novo, S; Muratori, I; et al. Women and peripheral arterial disease: same disease, different issues. *J Cardiovasc Med (Hagerstown)*, 2008, 9,382-8.

[128] Postley, JE; Perez, A; Wong, ND; Gardin, JM. Prevalence and distribution of sub-clinical atherosclerosis by screening vascular ultrasound in low and intermediate risk adults: the New York physicians study. *J Am Soc Echocardiogr*, 2009, 22,1145-51.

[129] Mazzeffi, MA; Lin, HM; Flynn, BC; O'Connell, TL; Delaet, DE. Hypothyroidism and the risk of lower extremity arterial disease. *Vasc Health Risk Manag*, 2010, 6,957-62.

[130] Paquet, M; Pilon, D; Tetrault, JP; Carrier, N. Protective vascular treatment of patients with peripheral arterial disease: guideline adherence according to year, age and gender. *Can J Public Health*, 2010, 101,96-100.

[131] Klein-Weigel, PF; Gutsche-Petrak, B; Wolbergs, S; Koning, C; Flessenkamper, I. Secondary medical prevention in patients with peripheral arterial disease - prescriptions of vascular surgeons and medical doctors (angiologists) in a multidisciplinary vascular centre. *Vasa*, 2010, 39,145-52.

[132] Rossouw, JE; Anderson, GL; Prentice, RL; LaCroix, AZ; Kooperberg, C; Stefanick, ML; et al. Risks and benefits of estrogen plus progestin in healthy postmenopausal women: Principal results From the Women's Health Initiative randomized controlled trial. *JAMA*, 2002, 288,321-33.

[133] Grady, D; Herrington, D; Bittner, V; Blumenthal, R; Davidson, M; Hlatky, M; et al. Cardiovascular disease outcomes during 6.8 years of hormone therapy, Heart and Estrogen/progestin Replacement Study follow-up (HERS II). *JAMA*, 2002, 288,49-57.

[134] Hsia, J; Simon, JA; Lin, F; Applegate, WB; Vogt, MT; Hunninghake, D; et al. Peripheral arterial disease in randomized trial of estrogen with progestin in women with coronary heart disease: The Heart and Estrogen/Progestin Replacement Study. *Circulation*, 2000, 102,2228-32.

[135] Hirsch, AT; Criqui, MH; Treat-Jacobson, D; Regensteiner, JG; Creager, MA; Olin, JW; et al. Peripheral arterial disease detection, awareness, and treatment in primary care. *JAMA*, 2001, 286,1317-24.

[136] Feinglass, J; McDermott, MM; Foroohar, M; Pearce, WH. Gender differences in interventional management of peripheral vascular disease: evidence from a blood flow laboratory population. *Ann Vasc Surg*, 1994, 8,343-9.

[137] McDermott, MM; Fried, L; Simonsick, E; Ling, S; Guralnik, JM. Asymptomatic peripheral arterial disease is independently associated with impaired lower extremity functioning: the women's health and aging study. *Circulation*, 2000, 101,1007-12.

[138] Oka, RK; Szuba, A; Giacomini, JC; Cooke, JP. Gender differences in perception of PAD: a pilot study. *Vasc Med*, 2003, 8,89-94.

[139] Cherr, GS; Wang, J; Zimmerman, PM; Dosluoglu, HH. Depression is associated with worse patency and recurrent leg symptoms after lower extremity revascularization. *J Vasc Surg*, 2007, 45,744-50.

[140] Selvin, E; Erlinger, TP. Prevalence of and risk factors for peripheral arterial disease in the United States: results from the National Health and Nutrition Examination Survey, 1999-2000. *Circulation*, 2004, 110,738-43.

[141] Bild, DE; Bluemke, DA; Burke, GL; Detrano, R; ez Roux, AV; Folsom, AR; et al. Multi-ethnic study of atherosclerosis:objectives and design. *Am J Epidemiol*, 2002, 156,871-81.

[142] Fowkes, FG; Murray, GD; Butcher, I; Heald, CL; Lee, RJ; Chambless, LE; et al. Ankle brachial index combined with Framingham Risk Score to predict cardiovascular events and mortality: a meta-analysis. *JAMA*, 2008, 300,197-208.

[143] Lonn, E; Roccaforte, R; Yi, Q; Dagenais, G; Sleight, P; Bosch, J; et al. Effect of long-term therapy with ramipril in high-risk women. *J Am CollCardiol*, 2002, 40,693-702.

[144] Herrington, DM; Vittinghoff, E; Lin, F; Fong, J; Harris, F; Hunninghake, D; et al. Statin therapy, cardiovascular events; and total mortality in the Heart and Estrogen/Progestin Replacement Study (HERS). *Circulation*, 2002, 105,2962-7.

[145] Sigvant, B; Wiberg-Hedman, K; Bergqvist, D; Rolandsson, O; Wahlberg, E. Risk factor profiles and use of cardiovascular drug prevention in women and men with peripheral arterial disease. *Eur J Cardiovasc Prev Rehabil*, 2009, 16,39-46.

[146] Cheanvechai, V; Harthun, NL; Graham, LM; Freischlag, JA; Gahtan, V. Incidence of peripheral vascular disease in women, is it different from that in men? *J Thorac Cardiovasc Surg*, 2004, 127,314-7.

[147] Ah Chong, AK; Chiu, KM; Wong, M; Yip, AW. The influence of gender difference on the outcomes of infrainguinal bypass for critical limb ischaemia in Chinese patients. *Eur J Vasc Endovasc Surg*, 2002, 23,134-9.

[148] Nguyen, LL; Hevelone, N; Rogers, SO; Bandyk, DF; Clowes, AW; Moneta, GL; et al. Disparity in outcomes of surgical revascularization for limb salvage: race and gender are synergistic determinants of vein graft failure and limb loss. *Circulation*, 2009, 119,123-30.

[149] Timaran, CH; Stevens, SL; Freeman, MB; Goldman, MH. Infrainguinal arterial reconstructions in patients with aortoiliac occlusive disease: the influence of iliac stenting. *J Vasc Surg*, 2001, 34,971-8.

[150] Hsia, J; Aragaki, A; Bloch, M; LaCroix, AZ; Wallace, R. Predictors of angina pectoris versus myocardial infarction from the Women's Health Initiative Observational Study. *Am J Cardiol*, 2004, 93,673-8.

[151] Hsia J; Criqui MH; Herrington DM; Manson JE; Wu L; Heckbert SR; et al. Conjugated equine estrogens and peripheral arterial disease risk: The Women's Health Initiative. *Am Heart J*, 2006,152,170-6.

[152] Hulley, S; Grady, D; Bush, T; Furberg, C; Herrington, D; Riggs, B; et al. Randomized trial of estrogen plus progestin for secondary prevention of coronary heart disease in postmenopausal women. Heart and Estrogen/progestin Replacement Study (HERS) Research Group. *JAMA*, 1998, 280,605-13.

[153] Mazhari, R; Hsia, J. Prevalence, clinical significance, and management of peripheral arterial disease in women: is there a role for postmenopausal hormone therapy? *Vasc Health Risk Manag*, 2005, 1,111-7.

[154] Magnant, JG; Cronenwett, JL; Walsh, DB; Schneider, JR; Besso, SR; Zwolak, RM. Surgical treatment of infrainguinal arterial occlusive disease in women. *J Vasc Surg*, 1993, 17,67-76.

[155] Mays, BW; Towne, JB; Fitzpatrick, CM; Smart, SC; Cambria, RA; Seabrook, GR; et al. Women have increased risk of perioperative myocardial infarction and higher long-term mortality rates after Surg, 1999, 29,807-12.

[156] Vouyouka, AG; Egorova, NN; Salloum, A; Kleinman, L; Marin, M; Faries, PL; et al. Lessons learned from the analysis of gender effect on risk factors and procedural outcomes of lower extremity arterial disease. *J Vasc Surg*, 2010, 52,1196-202.

BIOGRAPHICAL SKETCH

Name: PARLOOP AMIT BHATT

Affiliation: L. M. College of Pharmacy, Ahmedabad, India

Education: B.Pharm.,M.Pharm.(Pharmacology),PH.D, Diploma in Business Management(DBM)

Research and Professional Experience: Since 1987 (29 years) professionally involved in research

Professional Appointments

- Serving at L.M. College of Pharmacy since 1987 as a full time permanent faculty (Associate Professor).
- A Gujarat Technological University recognized M.Pharm(51) and PhD(4) guide in Pharmacology.
- Examiner at various universities at graduate and post graduate level.
- Ethics Committee member/chairperson reviewing pre-clinical (CPCSCEA) and clinical global trials at reputed Clinical Organizations.
- Data safety monitoring board committee member of a CRO.
- Reviewer/editorial board member for various national/ international journals like Diabetes, Obesity and metabolism; Dove Press Publications,Hindwai Publications,Indian Journal of Pharmacology,Journal of pharmacy and pharmacology, etc.

Honors

- Researched, Authored and Published (89) research articles in National (29) and International Journals (60), besides authored 2 books and 3 book chapters.
- Researched, Authored and presented (61) research articles at National (36)and International(25) conferences.
- Attended CME's, refresher courses, workshops and symposiums national and international conferences (49).
- Received recognitions from national and international organisations (31).
- Received Grants and sponsorships in vocational areas
- Guest Faculty/Speaker at number of Institutes, CME's, and Scientific meets.

Publications (last 3 years)

No	*Title*	*Vol./ Page No./ Year*	*Name of Journal*	*National/ International and ISSN No.*
1.	NCDR® as a Resource to Develop Cardiac Disease Specific Clinical Care Clinics	2016	Journal of American College of Cardiology	ISSN: 0735-1097 Proc.
2.	Hospital to Home Visit an Effective Health Care Initiative to Reduce Complications and Improve Drug Compliance and Adherence: NCDR® Participation Advantage	2016	Journal of American College of Cardiology	ISSN: 0735-1097 Proc.
3.	Real-World Safety and OutcomeMeasures of Novel Sirolimus Coated Balloon Catheter	2016	Journal of American College of Cardiology	ISSN: 0735-1097 Proc.
4.	Chest Pain in Acute Coronary Syndrome Patients with Depression after Bypass Surgery	2016	Catherization and cardiovascular therapy	ISSN: 1522-726X Proc.
5.	Effect of Mono-therapy versus Combinational Therapy on Exercise Capacity of Pulmonary Arterial Hypertension Patients: Actual Care Data	2016	Catherization and cardiovascular therapy	ISSN: 1522-726X Proc.
6.	Temporal Trends in Young Indian Heart Failure Patients: A Ray of Hope.	2016	Catherization and cardiovascular therapy	ISSN: 1522-726X Proc.
7.	Depression Adversely Affects Long Term Outcomes in Acute Coronary Syndrome Patients: A Real World Scenario	2016	Catherization and cardiovascular therapy	ISSN: 1522-726X Proc.
8.	An Asian IndianSingleCentreRadialAccessPercutaneous CoronaryIntervention Experience: NCDR® Findings	2016	Journal of American College of Cardiology	ISSN: 0735-1097,Proc.
9.	Unique Aspects of Coronary Artery Disease in Indian Women. DOI: 10.1007/s10557-015-6594-5	Aug;29(4):369-76, 2015	Cardiovascular Drugs and Therapy	ISSN: 0920-3206 ISSN: 1573-7241
10.	Prevalence of Cardiovascular Disease in India: Hype or Hope.	VOL -2/ 2015	Catherization and cardiovascular therapy	ISSN: 1522-726X Proc.

No	*Title*	*Vol./ Page No./ Year*	*Name of Journal*	*National/ International and ISSN No.*
11.	Long-term Safety and Performance of the Orbital Atherectomy System for Treating Calcified Coronary Artery Lesions: 5-Year Follow-Up in the ORBIT I Trial;DOI:10.1016/j.carrev.2015.03.007	2015 Jun;16(4): 213-6. Epub 2015 Mar 31	Cardiovascular revascularization medicine	ISSN:1553-8389
12.	Depression and outcome of patients with acute coronary syndrome: a 3 year follow-up study DOI:10.1016/S0735-1097(15)61383-3	Vol:65 (10-S)/ 03/2015	Journal of the American College of Cardiology	ISSN: 0735-1097
13.	Comparative safety and efficacy evaluation of ivabradine, metoprolol and its combination in management of inappropriate sinus tachycardia in coronary artery bypass graft patients	VOL:63 (12):A1569/ APRIL 2014	Journal of the American College of Cardiology	ISSN: 0735-1097 Proc.
14.	Prevalence, Assessment and Clinical Outcome in Cardiovascular Disease: Impact of Gender Disparities.	Volume 2(8)/4/ Aug 2014	Austin J Pharmacol Ther	ISSN: 2373-6208
15.	Comparative Evaluation of Safety Outcomes of Different Prosthetic Valves in Indian Subjects: Research and Reviews	Volume 2/July - September , 2014	Journal of Pharmacology and Toxicological studies,	e-ISSN: 2322-0139 p-ISSN: 2322-0120
16.	Orbital atherectomy system in treating calcified coronary lesions:3year follow up in first human use study (Orbit I trial).	Vol:15 (4)/204-208/6/ 2014	Cardiovascular revascularization medicine: including molecular interventions	ISSN:0920-3206
17.	Comparative safety and efficacy evaluation of Ivabradine, Metoprolol and its combination in management of Inappropriate Sinus Tachycardia in Coronary Artery Bypass Graft Patients.	Volume 63/ March 29 2014	J. of American College of Cardiology	ISSN: 0735-1097
18.	A Prospective Study to Evaluate Correlation between Coronary Heart Disease and Depression and Its Influence on Quality of Life and Clinical Outcomes	Vol:61/ March 12 2013	J. of American College of Cardiology	ISSN: 0735-1097

Review Articles (last 3 years)

Sr. No.	*Title*	*Vol./Page No/year*	*Name of Journal*	*National/ International and ISSN No.*
1.	Cardiovascular Disease in India-A Fact Sheet. Pharmaceutical Industry; Vision 2025	204-212/ 2014	Comprehensive forecast on Pharmaceutical Industry	National
2.	Coenzyme Q10 supplement in breast cancer: The nutrient on horizon	Volume 1/ 150-158/ June 2014	International Journal of Research in Multidiscipline	International ISSN: 2349 – 4875
3.	Being of a clinical pharmacist: Expectations and outcomes.	Vol:14/ Jan 2014	Editorial: Indian journal of pharmacology	International. ISSN: 0253-7613

In: Coronary Artery Disease
Editor: Courtney Burke
ISBN: 978-1-63485-330-9

Chapter 4

ROLE OF MULTI-DETECTOR COMPUTED TOMOGRAPHY IN THE DETECTION OF SUBCLINICAL CORONARY ATHEROSCLEROSIS IN PATIENTS WITHOUT KNOWN CORONARY ARTERY DISEASE

Kohichiro Iwasaki*, MD
Department of Cardiology,
Okayama Kyokuto Hospital, Okayama, Japan

ABSTRACT

Coronary artery disease (CAD) is a leading cause of mortality and morbidity worldwide. In approximately half of the patients with newly diagnosed CAD, the first presentation is either acute myocardial infarction or sudden cardiac death. Moreover, approximately half of those developing CAD have been classified as having low or intermediate risk on the basis of a current risk algorithm. Recent studies have demonstrated that the major determinant of risk for atherosclerotic cardiovascular disease in asymptomatic adults is the presence of the underlying disease

* Address for correspondence: Kohichiro Iwasaki, MD, Department of Cardiology, Okayama Kyokuto Hospital, 567-1, Kurata, Naka-ku. Okayama, Japan, TEL +81-86-276-3231, FAX +81-86-274-1028, E-mail; kiwasaki@kyokuto.or.jp.

itself, namely subclinical atherosclerosis. Thus, it is essential to detect subclinical CAD before the manifestation of clinical CAD events.

Multi-detector computed tomography (MDCT) is a promising modality to evaluate CAD. MDCT has an excellent capacity to detect hemodynamically relevant stenosis and vulnerable plaque (also called high-risk plaque). Thus, we reviewed the studies that investigated the prevalence and characteristics of CAD in patients without known CAD by using MDCT.

These studies demonstrated that the prevalence of subclinical CAD in asymptomatic patients with low to intermediate risk was high, and that a substantial number of patients had significant stenosis. On the other hand, the prevalence of non-calcified plaque in asymptomatic patients with no or mild coronary calcium was relatively low, and significant coronary stenosis was rare in these patients.

Among diabetic patients, approximately two-thirds had subclinical CAD. The prevalence of significant stenosis and high-risk plaque, namely high-risk CAD, was significantly higher in these patients compared with that in those without diabetes. Moreover, some clinical characteristics could predict diabetic patients with high-risk CAD. In stroke patients, approximately two-thirds had subclinical CAD and one-fifth had high-risk CAD. The prevalence of high-risk CAD was two-fold higher in stroke patients compared with that in non-stroke patients. Patients with mild to moderate chronic kidney disease (CKD) had higher prevalence of significant stenosis and coronary plaque than did those without CKD. However the prevalence of high-risk plaque was not significantly different between the two groups. About three-quarters of patients with carotid artery disease had subclinical CAD, and higher intima-media thickness was associated with high-risk CAD.

Statin treatment is a mainstay of the treatment of patients with CAD. However, our study showed that CAD and carotid artery disease progressed significantly despite normal lipid values due to standard statin therapy in asymptomatic patients without known CAD. This suggests that more intense lipid lowering will be needed to prevent progression of CAD and carotid artery disease.

Taken together, these studies suggest that MDCT can detect subclinical CAD in patients with low to intermediate risk of but without known CAD, and that subclinical CAD is highly prevalent. The prevalence of high-risk CAD is particularly high in patients with diabetes, stroke, CKD, and carotid artery disease, but without known CAD. Intensive statin therapy is needed to prevent the progression of subclinical coronary atherosclerosis.

Coronary artery disease (CAD) is a leading cause of mortality and morbidity in developing and developed countries [1]. In approximately 50% of patients with newly diagnosed CAD, the first presentation is either acute myocardial infarction or sudden cardiac death [2, 3]. In addition, approximately half of those developing CAD have been classified as having low or intermediate risk on the basis of a current risk algorithm [4-7]. Recent studies have demonstrated that the major determinant of risk for atherosclerotic cardiovascular disease in asymptomatic adults is the presence of the underlying disease itself, namely subclinical atherosclerosis [8]. Subclinical atherosclerosis represents the vascular memory of risk factor exposure [9]. Thus, it is essential to detect subclinical coronary atherosclerosis before the manifestation of clinical CAD events. There is a growing need for non-invasive imaging to detect subclinical atherosclerosis.

Multi-detector computed tomography (MDCT) is a promising modality to evaluate CAD. MDCT has an excellent capacity to detect hemodynamically relevant stenosis and vulnerable plaque (also called high-risk plaque). In this article, we review the MDCT studies that investigated the prevalence and characteristics of CAD in patients without known CAD.

MDCT offers two ways of assessing coronary atherosclerosis. When performed without a contrast agent, coronary calcium can be detected and quantified (coronary calcium score). When performed with a contrast agent, coronary plaques can be detected (coronary computed tomographic angiography).

Non-Contrast-Enhanced MDCT

Coronary Calcium Score (CCS)

The amount of calcium is quantified by using the so-called Agatston score [10]. The Agatston score calculates the calcium burden by multiplying the area of the calcified lesion by a weighting factor dependent on the peak signal of the lesion. Volume and mass scores are alternative methods to quantify coronary calcium; however, they are not widely used.

Coronary artery calcification signifies the presence of coronary atherosclerosis, and a strong linear correlation exists between total coronary artery atherosclerotic plaque burden and the extent of coronary artery calcification [11-14]. Coronary artery calcification has been found to be the most powerful predictor of cardiac events, providing independent and incremental information over risk factor-based assessment of asymptomatic patients [15, 16]. Patients without detectable calcium have a very low rate of coronary death or myocardial infarction (0.4%) over 3 to 5 years of observation [17-20]. A CCS <100, 100–400, and >400 usually defines low-, intermediate-, and high-risk groups, respectively (Figure 1).

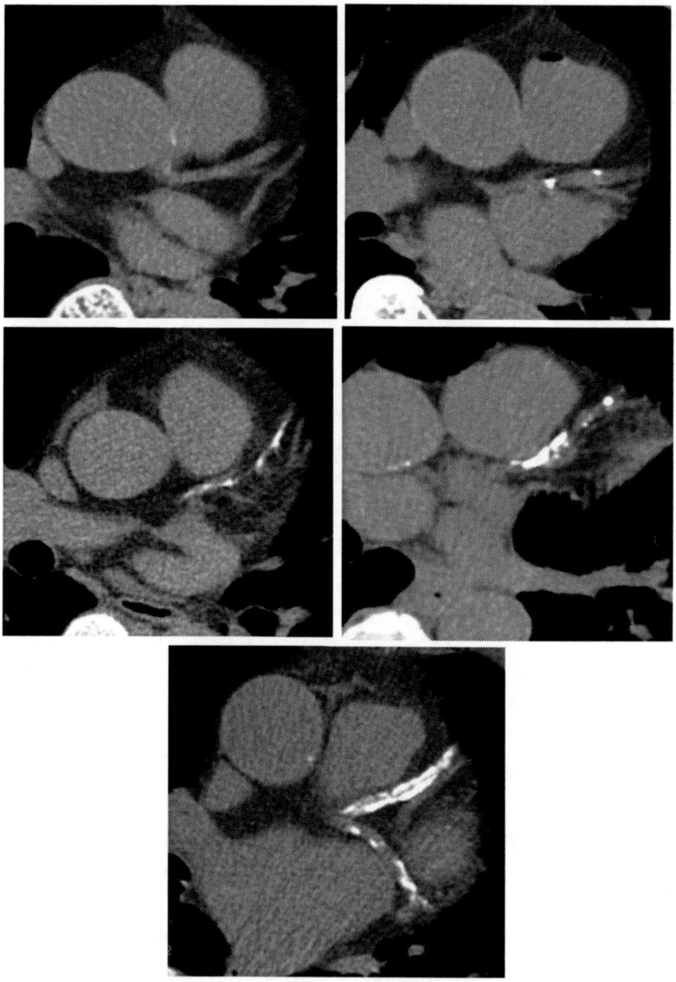

Figure 1. Representative cases of coronary calcium score. A: Coronary calcium score of 0. B: Coronary calcium score of 34. C: Coronary calcium score of 258. D: Coronary calcium score of 424. E: Coronary calcium score of 2,892.

Coronary Computed Tomographic Angiography (CCTA)

With 64-slice MDCT and adequate patient preparation, previous studies have reported rates of sensitivity ranging from 91% to 99% and specificity between 93% and 98% for the detection of hemodynamically relevant stenosis, in comparison with coronary angiography [21-24]. Thus, the diagnostic accuracy of CCTA has already been definitively established. In well-performed, prospective multicenter studies, CCTA is an accurate diagnostic modality with superior accuracy to detect and exclude anatomically obstructive CAD [25-27]. Furthermore, its ability to detect and characterize coronary plaques is well recognized [28-32]. In studies that compared MDCT with intravascular ultrasound, sensitivities and specificities for the detection of coronary artery segments with plaque have been reported to be between 80% and 90% [28, 29, 31].

Generally, most coronary events are caused by significant stenosis or vulnerable plaque. Many studies have demonstrated that significant stenosis increased the risk of future coronary events [33, 34]. Recent studies have also demonstrated that 70–80% of cardiac deaths and myocardial infarctions are caused by rupture of vulnerable plaques, which often present with non-significant stenosis [35, 36].

Significant Stenosis

Many studies have demonstrated that significant stenosis is associated with coronary events, and the increasing incidence of significant stenosis is associated with more coronary events [33, 34]. Patients with non-significant stenosis are at an increased risk of coronary events compared with those with normal coronary arteries, but have a more favorable prognosis compared with those with significant stenosis. Usually, significant or obstructive stenosis is defined as ≧50% diameter stenosis, and non-significant or non- obstructive stenosis is defined as <50% diameter stenosis (Figure 2 and 3).

In the CONFIRM (Coronary CT Angiography Evaluation for Clinical Outcomes: An International Multicenter) registry, 24,775 patients without known CAD who underwent CCTA were followed for 2.3 ± 1.1 years [33]. Both per-patient obstructive (hazard ratio [HR] 2.60, 95% confidence interval [CI] 1.94–3.49, $p < 0.0001$) and non-obstructive (HR 1.60, 95% CI 1.18–2.16, $p = 0.002$) CAD conferred increased risk of mortality compared with that in patients without evident CAD. Incident mortality was associated with a dose-response relationship to the number of coronary vessels exhibiting obstructive CAD, with increasing risk observed for non-obstructive (HR 1.62, 95% CI 1.20–2.19, $p = 0.002$), obstructive 1-vessel (HR 2.00, 95% CI 1.43–2.82, $p < 0.0001$), 2-vessel (HR 2.92, 95% CI 2.00–4.25, $p < 0.0001$), or 3-vessel or left main (HR 3.70, 95% CI 2.58–5.29, $p < 0.0001$) CAD. Importantly, the absence of CAD, as revealed by CCTA, was associated with a low rate of incident death (annualized death rate: 0.28%).

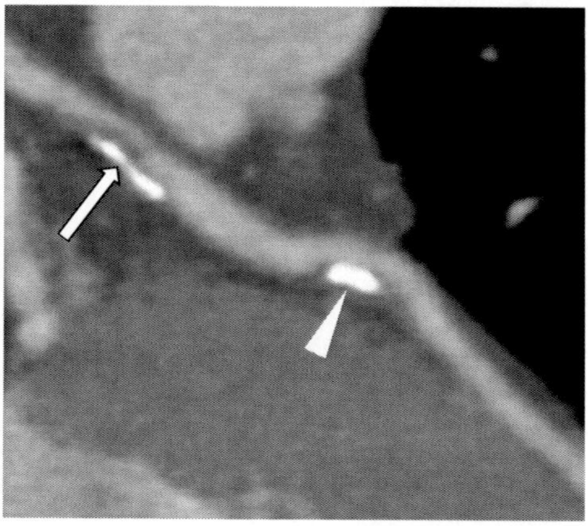

Figure 2. Significant and non-significant stenosis. Significant stenosis (arrow) in the proximal portion and non-significant stenosis (arrow head) in the distal portion of the left anterior descending coronary artery.

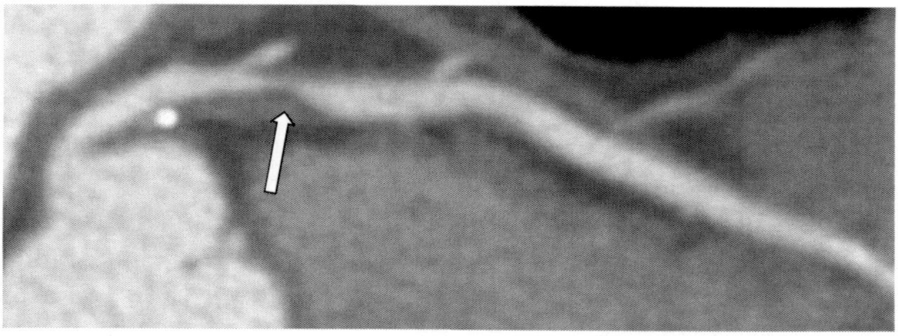

Figure 3. Significant stenosis. Significant stenosis in the proximal portion of the left anterior descending coronary artery.

Bamber et al. [37] performed a meta-analysis using 11 eligible articles including 7,335 participants with suspected CAD. The presence of ≥1 significant coronary stenosis was associated with an annualized event rate of

11.9%. The estimated HRs for left main stenosis, presence of plaque, and each coronary segment containing plaque were 6.64 (95% CI: 2.6–17.3), 4.51 (95% CI: 2.2–9.3), and 1.23 (95% CI: 1.17–1.29), respectively. Hulten et al. [38] performed another meta-analysis using 18 studies that evaluated 9,592 patients with a median follow-up of 20 months. The pooled annualized event rate for obstructive CAD versus normal CCTA was 8.8% versus 0.17% per year for major adverse cardiac events (MACE, $p < 0.05$) and 3.2% versus 0.15% for death or MI ($p < 0.05$). The pooled negative likelihood ratio for MACE after normal CCTA finding was 0.008 (95% CI 0.0004–0.17, $p < 0.001$), the positive likelihood ratio was 1.70 (95% CI 1.42–2.02, $p < 0.001$), the sensitivity was 0.99 (95% CI 0.93–1.00, $p < 0.001$), and the specificity was 0.41 (95% CI 0.31–0.52, $p < 0.001$). Stratifying by the absence of CAD, non-obstructive CAD, or obstructive CAD, incremental adverse events were observed.

Taken together, these studies demonstrate that the presence and extent of coronary stenosis on CCTA are strong independent predictors of cardiovascular events.

Vulnerable Plaque

Vulnerable plaque is often called high-risk plaque in the field of CT. High-risk plaque is defined as plaque with positive remodeling (PR), low attenuation, spotty calcification, or a napkin-ring sign. PR is defined as a diameter at the plaque site more than 10% larger than that of a reference segment [39] (Figure 4). Low-attenuation plaque (LAP) is defined as the lowest CT number of five areas of minimum region of interest less than 30 Hounsfield units (HU) in non-calcified plaque or plaque with spotty calcification [39] (Figure 5). Spotty calcification is defined as a calcification <3 mm in size on curved multiplanar reformation images and occupies only one side on cross-sectional images [39] (Figure 5). A napkin-ring sign is usually defined as the presence of a ring of high attenuation around certain coronary artery plaque, with CT attenuation of the ring presenting higher than that of adjacent plaque but no greater than 130 HU [40] (Figure 6).

Motoyama et al. [39] performed CCTA in 38 patients with acute coronary syndrome (ACS) and 33 patients with stable angina pectoris (SAP) before percutaneous coronary intervention. They found that PR (87% vs. 12%, $p < 0.0001$), LAP (79% vs. 9%, $p < 0.0001$), and spotty calcification (63% vs. 21%, $p = 0.0005$) were significantly more frequent in ACS lesions. The presence of all three showed a high positive predictive value, and the absence of all three showed a high negative predictive value for the culprit plaques associated with ACS.

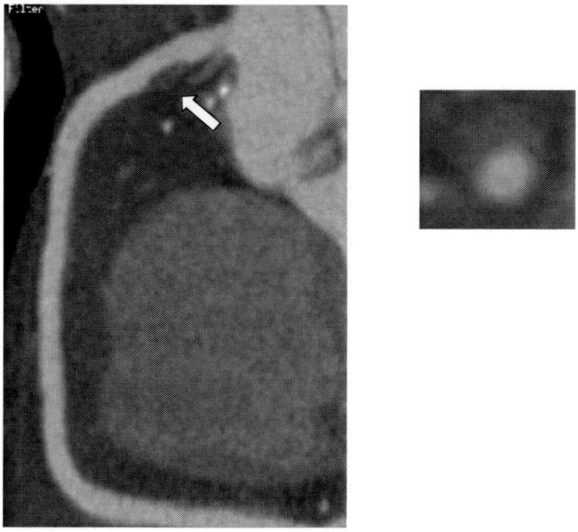

Figure 4. Positive remodeling. Positive remodeling was shown in the proximal portion of the right coronary artery.

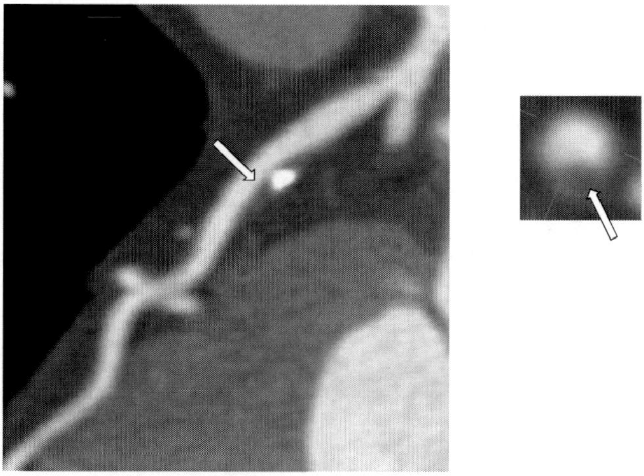

Figure 5. Positive remodeling, low attenuation plaque, and spotty calcification. Positive remodeling, low attenuation plaque, and spotty calcification were found in the proximal portion of the left anterior descending coronary artery.

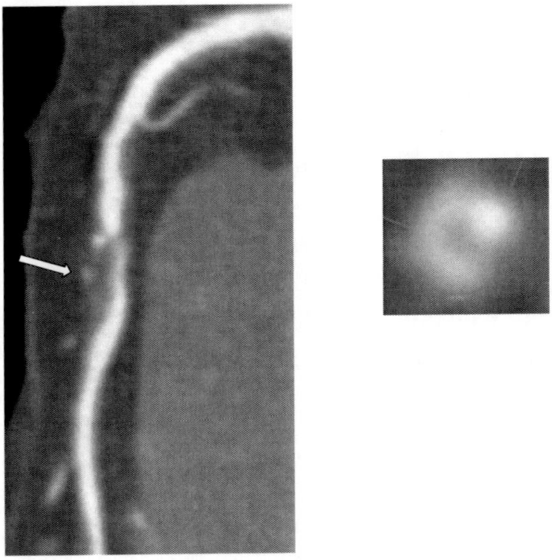

Figure 6. Napkin-ring sign. Napkin-ring sign was shown in the middle portion of the right coronary artery.

The same authors [41] followed 1,059 patients who underwent CCTA for a mean period of 27±10 months. Of the 45 patients showing plaques with both PR and LAP (two-feature positive plaques), ACS developed in 10 (22.2%), compared with 1 (3.7%) of the 27 patients with plaques displaying either feature (one-feature positive plaques). ACS developed in only 4 (0.5%) of the 820 patients with neither PR nor LAP (two-feature negative plaques). None of the 167 patients with normal angiograms had acute coronary events ($p < 0.001$). ACS was independently predicted by PR and/or LAP (HR 22.8, 95% CI 6.9–75.2, $p < 0.001$). Thus, patients demonstrating positively remodeled coronary segments with LAP were at a higher risk of ACS developing over time than those who had lesions without these characteristics.

Otsuka et al. [40] studied 895 consecutive patients who underwent CCTA examination and were followed for >1 year [38]. The CCTA analysis included the presence of obstructive plaque, PR, LAP, and a napkin-ring sign. During the follow-up period of 2.3 ± 0.8 years, 24 patients (2.6%) experienced ACS events. Segment-based Cox proportional hazards models analysis showed that PR ($p < 0.001$), LAP ($p = 0.007$), and the napkin-ring sign ($p < 0.0001$) were independent predictive factors for future ACS events.

Collectively, these studies demonstrate that these high-risk plaques are strongly and independently associated with ACS.

Subclinical Atherosclerosis

Prevalence and Prognosis

The PESA (Progression of Early Subclinical Atherosclerosis) study [42] enrolled 4,184 asymptomatic participants 40 to 54 years of age and evaluated the systemic extent of atherosclerosis in the carotid, abdominal aortic, and iliofemoral territories. The extent of subclinical atherosclerosis was classified as focal (one site affected), intermediate (two to three sites), or generalized (four to six sites). Subclinical atherosclerosis was present in 63% of participants. Plaques were most common in the iliofemorals (44%), followed by the carotids (31%), aorta (25%), and coronary arteries (18%). Among participants with a low Framingham Risk Score (FRS), subclinical disease was detected in 58%, with intermediate or generalized disease in 36%. Thus, subclinical atherosclerosis was highly prevalent in this middle-aged cohort, with nearly half of the participants classified as having intermediate or generalized disease.

The High Risk Plaque BioImage Study (A Clinical Study of Burden of Atherosclerotic Disease in an At-Risk Population) [43] investigated 6,101 asymptomatic persons without known cardiovascular disease and measured CCS, carotid intima-media thickness (IMT), ankle-brachial index (ABI), and abdominal aortic diameter (AAD). The mean age was 68.8 years, and 65.3% had intermediate FRS. Carotid plaques were identified in 78% of cases, abnormal ABI in 10%, AAD >20 mm in 28%, and coronary calcium in 68% of participants. Thus, the prevalence of subclinical atherosclerosis in an elderly cohort was much higher compared with a middle-aged cohort.

The BioImage Study [44] enrolled 5,808 asymptomatic adults (mean age 69 years, 56.5% female) and performed CCS measurement and novel 3-dimensional carotid ultrasound. Plaque areas from both carotid arteries were summed as the carotid plaque burden (cPB). Over a median follow-up of 2.7 years, MACE occurred in 216 patients (4.2%). Compared with individuals without any cPB, HR for MACE was 0.78 (95% CI 0.31–1.91), 1.45 (95% CI 0.67–3.14), and 2.36 (95% CI 1.13–4.92), respectively, with increasing cPB tertile, and with similar results for CCS. Thus, detection of subclinical carotid or coronary atherosclerosis improves risk predictions compared with conventional risk factors, with comparable results for either modality.

Subclinical Coronary Atherosclerosis in Patients with Low to Intermediate Risk

We [45] performed MDCT in 415 asymptomatic patients with coronary risk factors but without known CAD. The mean age was 67.4 ± 10.9 years. According to NIPPON DATA 80 [46], 194 (46.7%) patients were at low risk, 212 (51.1%) were at intermediate risk, and only 9 (2.2%) were at high risk. However, we detected coronary plaques in 295 patients (71.1%). Importantly, of 135 patients with CCS of zero, non-calcified plaques were detected in 15 (11.1%). A total of 235 patients (79.7%) had multiple plaques, with an average 4.6 plaques/patient. The CCS was zero in only 135 patients (32.5%) and CCS >400 was found in 76 (18.3%). Significant stenosis was detected in 91 patients (21.9%) and 85 underwent stress myocardial perfusion imaging. Myocardial ischemia was found in 27 patients (31.8%), and 21 (24.7%) underwent percutaneous coronary intervention. In a mean follow-up period of 2.8 years, four patients developed ACS. Thus, our results demonstrated that about 70% of asymptomatic patients with low to intermediate risk had subclinical CAD and one-fifth had significant stenosis.

One study [47] performed MDCT in 161 patients with intermediate risk for CAD. They found non-calcified plaques in 10 patients (6.2%) and calcified plaques in 98 (60.9%). Thus, the prevalence of coronary plaques was 67.1%. Their results are similar to ours. Another study [48] investigated 1,000 middle-aged asymptomatic subjects and identified atherosclerotic plaques in 215 (22%) individuals, of whom 40 (4%) had only non-calcified plaques. The prevalence was much lower compared with our study; the subjects were younger and far fewer had hypertension, hyperlipidemia, and diabetes, compared with our patients. Thus, these studies showed that subclinical CAD was highly prevalent in patients with low to intermediate risk but without known CAD.

Non-Calcified Coronary Plaque

We [49] studied 224 asymptomatic patients with zero CCS (no CCS group, n = 117) and those with mild CCS, defined as CCS 1–100 (mild CCS group, n = 107) (Figure 7). Patients of the no CCS group were younger and less often had diabetes compared with those of the mild CCS group. The prevalence of non-calcified plaque was 11.1% in the no CCS group and 23.4% in the mild CCS group ($p = 0.014$). Multiple plaques were detected in 2.6% and 3.7% ($p = 0.593$), respectively. Significant stenosis was found in one patient in the no CCS group (0.9%) and three patients in the mild CCS group (2.8%, $p = 0.351$).

Previous studies showed that the prevalence of non-calcified plaque in patients without coronary calcium was 6.5 to 15.9% [47, 50, 51]. These results are similar to ours. As for patients with mild coronary calcium, the prevalence of non-calcified plaque was 23.4% in our study. However the prevalence was 65.2% in Cheng's study [50] and 53.8% in Rubinshtein's study [52]. Our study patients represent a lower risk population than prior similar studies, hence the lower prevalence of non-calcified plaque.

As a whole, these results showed that significant percentages of non-calcified plaque were found in asymptomatic low risk patients with no or mild coronary calcium but that significant coronary stenosis was rare in these patients. Moreover, the finding of zero or low CCS does not guarantee good endothelial/coronary health, and such patients may still be at risk.

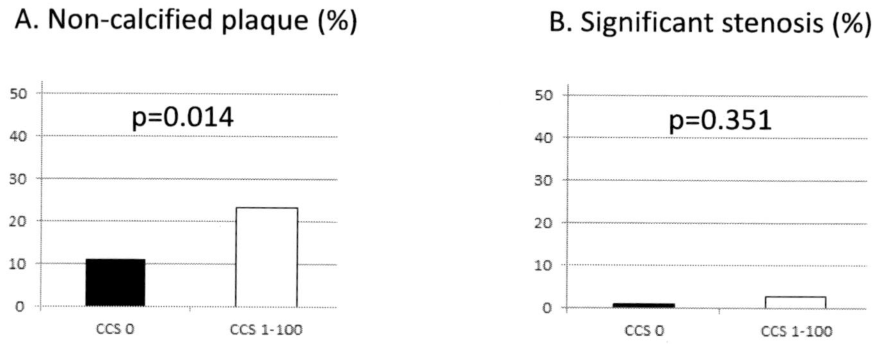

Figure 7. Non-calcified plaque. A: Prevalence of non-calcified plaque, B: Prevalence of significant stenosis. Modified from Iwasaki et al. [49].

Application and Efficacy of CCTA

Coronary Artery Disease

Distribution of Coronary Atherosclerosis

We [53] measured CCS in 624 consecutive patients for the right coronary artery (RCA), left main trunk (LMT), left anterior descending coronary artery (LAD), and left circumflex coronary artery (LCX), then calculated total CCS. We divided these patients into 4 groups: CCS 1-100 (Group A, n = 267), CCS 101-400 (Group B, n = 160), CCS 401-1,000 (Group C, n = 110), and CCS >1,000 (Group D, n = 87). In Group A, B, and C, the CCS in LAD was significantly higher than that in the other three arteries ($p < 0.0001$). In Group

D, the CCS was not significantly different between LAD and RCA (p = 0.693, Figure 8). This was also true for the prevalence of coronary calcium (Figure 9). Thus, coronary calcium was found more frequently in LAD than in the other coronary arteries in patients with mild to high CCS, but not in those with very high CCS.

Our study demonstrates the usefulness of topography of coronary calcium by MDCT in predicting the natural history of patients with variable degrees of coronary atherosclerosis. The LAD perfuses the broadest area of myocardium and ischemia in the LAD territory results in the most severe clinical consequences. The LAD is also the most frequent culprit artery in ischemic events [54-56].

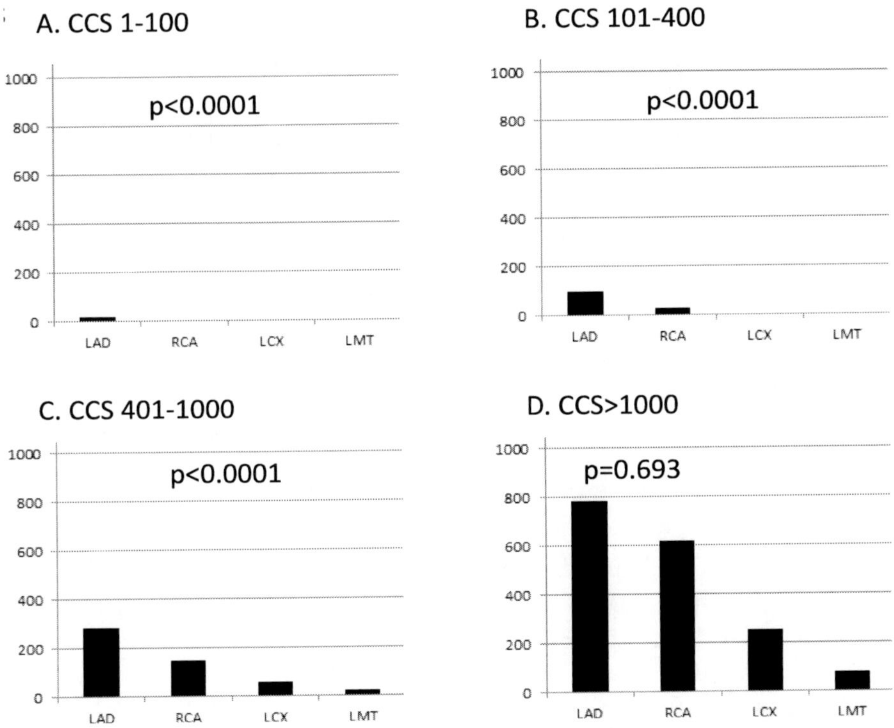

Figure 8. CCS in each coronary artery. Abbreviations: LAD; left anterior descending coronary artery, LCX; left circumflex coronary artery, LMT; left main trunk, RCA; right coronary artery. Modified from Iwasaki et al. [53].

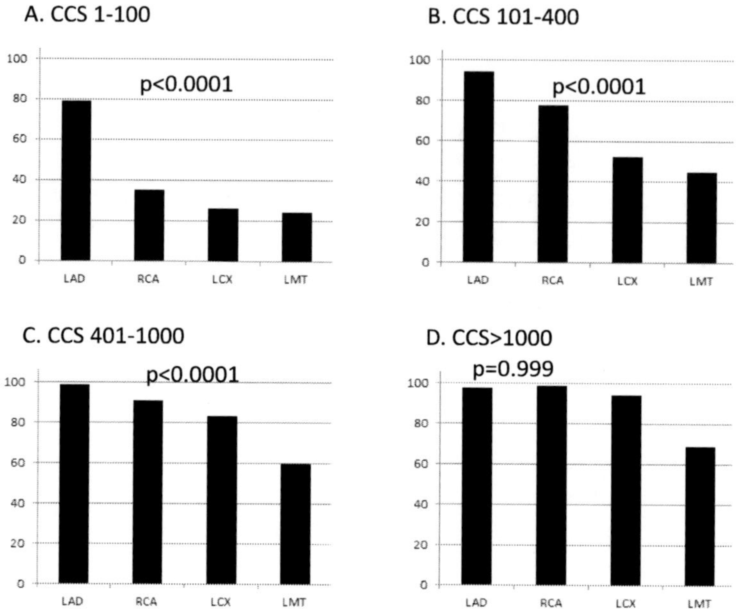

Figure 9. Prevalence of coronary calcium in each coronary artery. Abbreviations: the same as Figure 8. Modified from Iwasaki et al. (53).

Epicardial Fat

Epicardial fat (EF) is the visceral fat of the heart deposited under the visceral layer of the pericardium and has the same origin as abdominal visceral fat, which is shown to be strongly related to the development of CAD [57-59].

We [60] measured the volume of EF (EFV) by MDCT and studied the relationship between EFV and the severity of CAD in 197 patients (Figure 10). EFV was 99.4±40.0 (11.6 to 263.8) ml and CCS was 267.2±605.1 (0 to 3780). There was a significant but modest relationship between EFV and CCS ($r = 0.210$, $p = 0.003$). CCS was significantly higher in patients with EFV >100 than those with EFV <100 (median 75 vs. 23, $p = 0.016$). The incidence of significant stenosis was significantly higher in patients with EFV >100 compared with those with EFV <100 (40.2% vs. 22.7%, $p = 0.008$). The EFV and prevalence of EFV >100 were significantly higher in patients with severe coronary artery stenosis, defined as percent diameter stenosis of 70% to 90%, and in those with severe coronary artery calcification, defined as CCS >400. Thus, our results showed that EFV was associated with coronary atherosclerosis, and the EFV increased sharply in patients with severe coronary stenosis and those with severe coronary calcification.

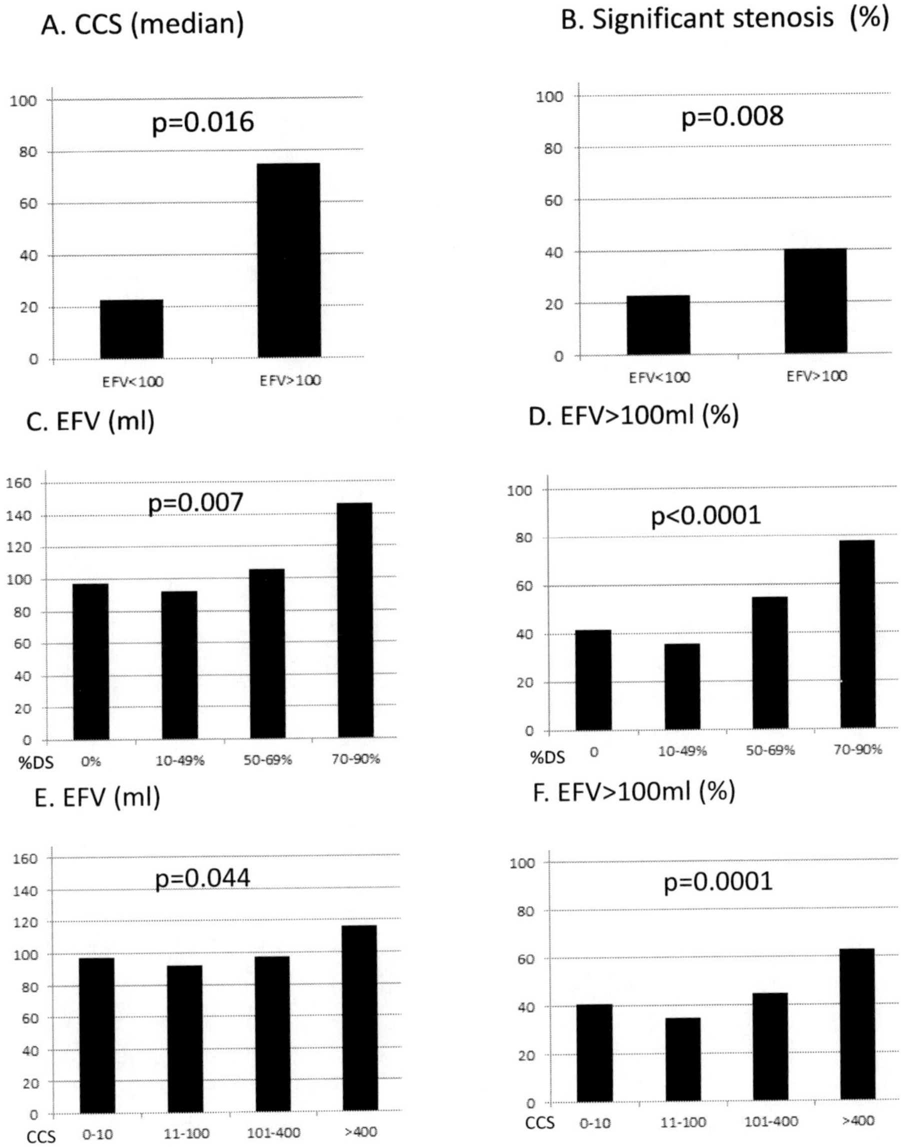

Figure 10. Epicardial fat volume (EFV). A: Median value of coronary calcium score (CCS), B: Prevalence of significant stenosis, C: Relationship between EFV and degree of coronary stenosis, D: Relationship between prevalence of EFV >100 ml and degree of coronary stenosis, E: Relationship between EFV and severity of coronary calcium, F: Relationship between prevalence of EFV >100 ml and severity of coronary calcium. Modified from Iwasaki et al. [60].

Although recent studies found a modest relationship between EFV and severity of CAD, most studies did not find a stepwise increase of EFV with increasing severity of coronary atherosclerosis. One study [61] found that EFV was not associated with severity of coronary atherosclerosis and the extent of coronary calcification, although such a relationship was found in patients with body mass index <27. Another study [62] found that EFV did not increase with increasing severity of atherosclerosis in spite of a significant correlation between EFV and the presence of coronary atherosclerosis. In contrast, our results showed that EFV was significantly higher only in patients with the most severe coronary stenosis and most severe coronary calcification. Ueno et al. [63] found that increased EFV was the strongest independent determinant of the presence of totally occluded lesions. Therefore, our results suggest that epicardial fat accumulation does not increase stepwise with increasing severity of coronary atherosclerosis, but increases sharply with the development of severe coronary stenosis and severe coronary calcification.

Diabetes Mellitus

Subclinical Coronary Atherosclerosis

Patients with type 2 diabetes have a two- to four-fold higher risk of a cardiovascular event than nondiabetic patients [64]. Previous studies have shown that the risk of myocardial infarction in a diabetic patient is comparable to the risk of recurrent infarction in a nondiabetic patient with a previous myocardial infarction [65]. Remarkably, 65% to 75% of diabetic patients die of cardiovascular disease [66].

We [67] studied 93 diabetic patients (diabetic group) and 93 age- and sex-matched non-diabetic patients without known CAD (non-diabetic group) (Figure 11). Clinical characteristics were not significantly different between the two groups. The CCS was significantly higher in the diabetic group than in the non-diabetic group (median 117 vs. 54, $p < 0.0001$). No coronary calcium was detected in 15.1% and 30.0% in the diabetic and non-diabetic groups, respectively ($p = 0.002$). CCS >400 was detected in 36.6% and 9.7% in each group ($p < 0.0001$). Coronary plaques were found in 91.4% and 67.7% in each group ($p < 0.0001$). Multiple plaques were detected in 77.4% and 57.0% in each group ($p = 0.003$). Significant coronary stenosis was found in 33.3% and 16.1% in each group ($p = 0.007$). Thus, our results showed that the prevalence of subclinical CAD in diabetic patients was very high.

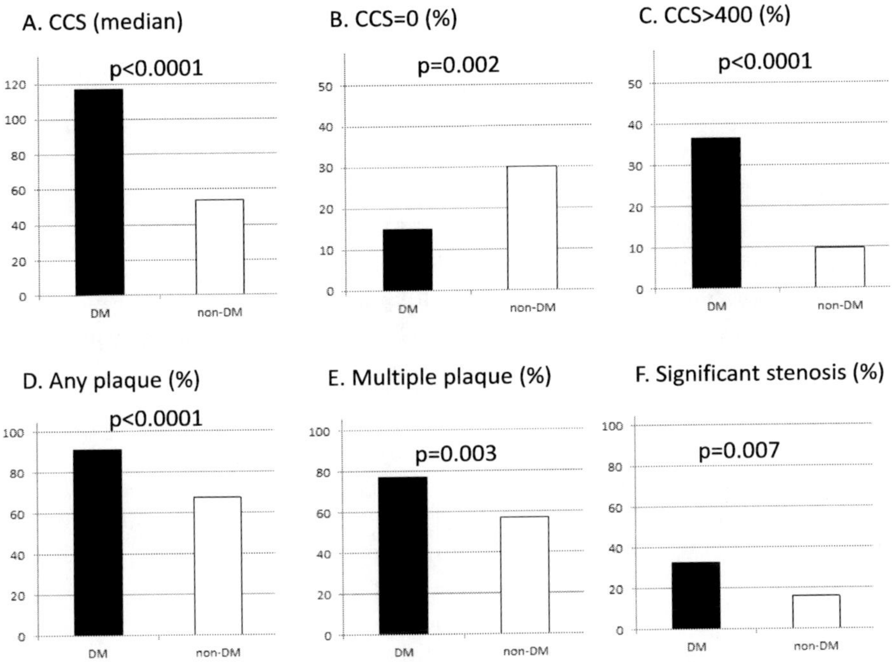

Figure 11. Diabetes mellitus. A: Median value of coronary calcium score (CCS), B: Prevalence of CCS of 0, C: Prevalence of CCS >400, D: Prevalence of any plaque, E: Prevalence of multiple plaques, F: Prevalence of significant stenosis. Modified from Iwasaki et al. [67].

One study [68] measured CCS in 155 asymptomatic diabetic patients and found that 72% had coronary calcium and 48% had a coronary calcium score >102. Another study [69] performed CCTA in 215 symptomatic patients (86 with diabetes), and found that diabetic patients showed significantly more diseased coronary segments with more non-obstructive plaques. Relatively more non-calcified and calcified and fewer mixed plaques were observed in diabetic patients. Maffei et al. [70] studied 1,126 patients without known CAD (147 with diabetes). Diabetic patients had a higher number of diseased segments, a higher rate of CCS ≧400, and obstructive CAD, and fewer normal coronary arteries as compared to non-diabetic patients. Furthermore, we [71] performed MDCT in 374 patients without known CAD. We divided the patients into those with diabetes (diabetes group, n = 138) and those without diabetes (non-diabetes group, n = 236). Patient characteristics were not significantly different between the two groups. The CCS was significantly higher in the diabetes group than the non-diabetes group (median 202 vs. 60, p

= 0.0002). The prevalence of significant stenosis (17.4% vs. 6.8%, p = 0.001) and coronary plaques (4.3±4.3 vs. 3.1±4.4, p = 0.009) was significantly higher in the diabetes group compared with the nondiabetes group. The prevalence of high-risk plaque (PR and LAP) was not significantly different between the two groups (9.4% vs. 9.7%, p = 0.92). However, in a multiple logistic regression analysis adjusted for variables associated with a high-risk plaque, only diabetes was significantly associated with a high-risk plaque.

Taken together, these studies showed that diabetic patients had more atherosclerotic plaque burden manifested by higher CCS, higher prevalence of significant stenosis, higher prevalence of calcified and non-calcified plaques, and higher prevalence of high-risk plaque compared with non-diabetic patients.

Detection of High-Risk CAD

As stated above, subclinical CAD is highly prevalent in diabetic patients without known CAD. However, the number of diabetic patients is huge and factors associated with high-risk CAD are not thoroughly studied.

We performed MDCT in 289 diabetic patients without known CAD [72]. We studied the factors associated with high-risk CCS, defined as CCS ≧400, significant stenosis, defined as percent diameter stenosis ≧50%, and high-risk plaque, defined as PR, LAP, spotty calcification, or a napkin-ring sign, using univariate and multivariate analysis. These analyses showed that the age (odds ratio [OR] 1.05/year, 95% CI 1.01–1.08, p = 0.0085), duration of diabetes (OR 1.06/year, 95% CI 1.02–1.10, p = 0.0020), and hypertension (OR 2.09, 95% CI 1.15–3.82, p = 0.016) were predictors of high-risk CCS. Hypertension (OR 3.58, 95% CI 1.42–9.03, p = 0.0069) was a predictor of significant stenosis. Dyslipidemia (OR 2.15, 95% CI 0.99–4.63, p = 0.0522) was marginally a predictor of significant stenosis. Male sex (OR 3.01, 95% CI 1.46–6.23, p = 0.0029) and duration of diabetes (OR 1.05/year, 95% CI 1.01–1.09, p = 0.0133) were predictors of high-risk plaque. Thus, our results showed that in diabetic patients without known CAD, age, male sex, duration of diabetes, and hypertension were predictors of high-risk CAD. These simple risk factors may guide the consideration of indications for CCTA in diabetic patients without known CAD.

Kim et al. [73] analyzed 933 asymptomatic diabetic patients without known CAD who underwent CCTA. Patients were divided into three groups according to the duration of diabetes: <5 years, 5-10 years, and ≥10 years. Patients with longer duration of diabetes had higher rates of obstructive CAD. Patients with longer duration of diabetes were associated with a higher prevalence, extent, and severity of CAD, as well as risk of major adverse cardiac and cerebrovascular events.

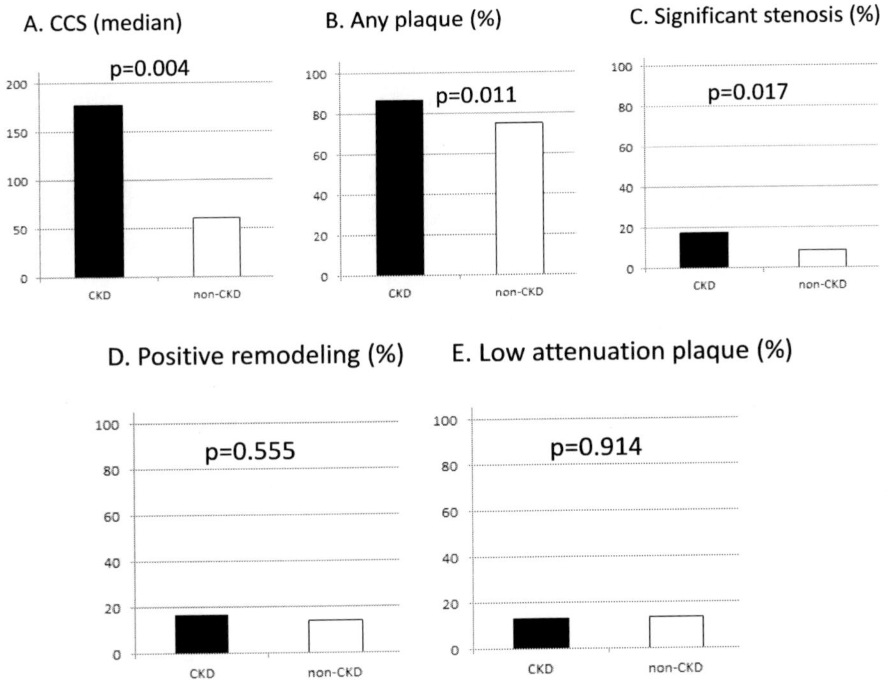

Figure 12. Chronic kidney disease. A: Median value of coronary calcium score (CCS), B: Prevalence of any plaque, C: Prevalence of significant stenosis, D: Prevalence of positive remodeling, E: Prevalence of low attenuation plaque.

Chronic Kidney Disease (CKD)

Subclinical Coronary Atherosclerosis

We performed CCTA in 347 patients without known CAD. We divided these patients into those with CKD (CKD group, n = 108) and those without CKD (non-CKD group, n = 239) (Figure 12). CKD was defined as estimated GFR 30-59 ml/min/1.73 m^2. Patients in the CKD group were older, more likely to be female, and had a higher prevalence of hypertension. The CCS was significantly higher in the CKD group than the non-CKD group (median 177 vs. 61, p = 0.004). The prevalence of coronary plaque (87.0% vs. 74.9%, p = 0.011) and significant stenosis (17.6% vs. 8.8%, p = 0.017) was significantly higher in the CKD group. However the prevalence of PR (16.7% vs. 14.2%, p = 0.555) and LAP (13.0% vs. 13.4%, p = 0.914) was not significantly different between the two groups. Thus, our results showed that patients with mild to moderate CKD had higher CCS, and higher prevalence of significant stenosis and coronary plaque compared with those without CKD. However, the prevalence of high-risk plaque was not significantly different between the two groups.

One study [74] performed CCTA in 313 patients and found that high CCS (>445) was significantly correlated with age, CKD, and number of diseased vessels. Another study [75] performed CCTA in 4,297 asymptomatic subjects and found that early CKD was an independent risk factor for CAD. However, neither the risk of CAD nor CCS >100 increased as stage of CKD advanced. There is only one study which focused on the characteristics of coronary plaque in patients with CKD. Kawai et al. [76] studied 487 patients with suspected stable CAD and found that the severity of coronary artery stenosis was higher in patients with mild CKD, although there was no significant difference in the prevalence of high-risk plaque. Their results are similar to ours.

Carotid Artery Disease

Subclinical Coronary Atherosclerosis

We [77] studied 100 asymptomatic patients with IMT >1.0 mm (Figure 13). We divided these patients into two groups according to a median value of maximum IMT. Coronary calcium was detected in 74.0% of patients and coronary plaque was detected in 77.0%. Median value of CCS was 21 and 140 in patients with maximum IMT <1.7 mm and >1.8 mm, respectively, (p = 0.003). No calcium was detected in 35.3% and 16.3% (p = 0.031), respectively. CCS >400 was found in 9.8% and 28.6% (p = 0.017), respectively. Median number of coronary plaques was three and six (p = 0.048) in each group. Prevalence of any plaque was 68.6% and 85.7% (p = 0.042) in each group. Significant stenosis was found in 29% of patients. Thus, our results showed that the prevalence of CAD in asymptomatic patients with carotid artery disease was very high, and that higher IMT was associated with higher CCS and higher prevalence of coronary plaque and significant stenosis.

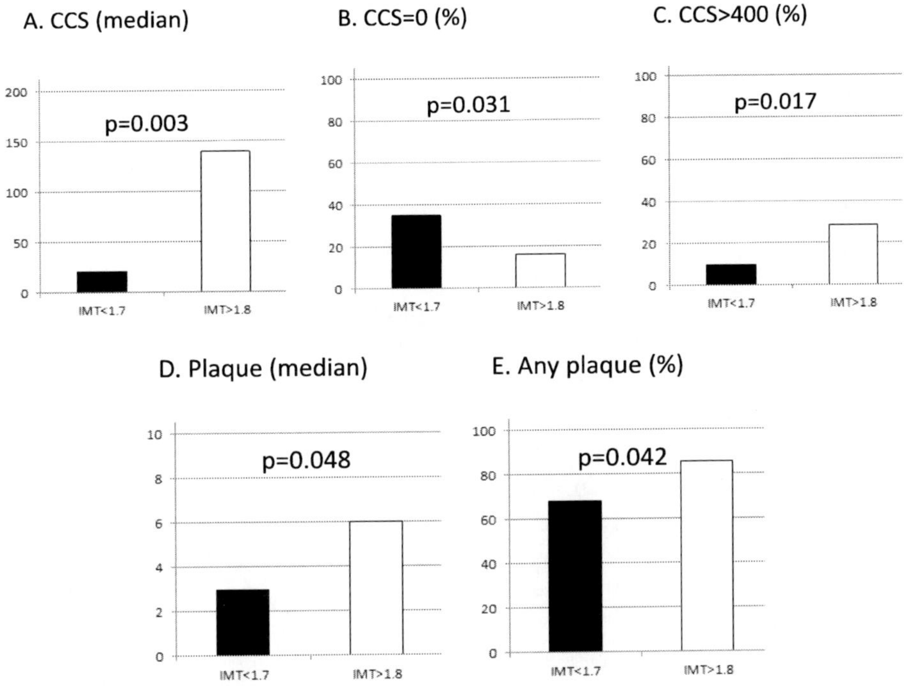

Figure 13. Carotid artery disease. A: Median value of coronary calcium score (CCS), B: Prevalence of CCS of 0, C: Prevalence of CCS >400, D: Median number of plaques, E: Prevalence of any plaque. Modified from Iwasaki et al. [77].

Carotid IMT correlates with the degree of carotid atherosclerosis measured at autopsy and has been found to correlate with atherosclerotic vascular disease in other arterial beds [78, 79]. Ultrasound-derived carotid IMT is considered a surrogate for systemic atherosclerotic disease burden [80].

IMT findings have been demonstrated to correlate with cardiac and cerebrovascular outcomes [81-83]. A meta-analysis [84] showed that the age- and sex-adjusted overall estimates of the relative risk of myocardial infarction were 1.26 per 1-standard deviation common carotid artery IMT difference and 1.15 per 0.10-mm common carotid artery IMT difference. In a substudy of the Cardiovascular Health Study, Newman et al. [85] found that internal carotid IMT was most closely related to coronary artery calcium.

Ischemic Stroke

Subclinical Coronary Atherosclerosis

Recently, ischemic stroke without carotid artery disease has emerged as a new coronary heart disease risk equivalent. An American Heart Association/ American Stroke Association Scientific Statement concludes that patients with atherosclerotic stroke should be included among those deemed to be at high risk (≥20% over 10 years) of further atherosclerotic coronary events [86].

We [87] measured CCS in 151 ischemic stroke patients without known CAD (stroke group) and compared the results with 151 age- and sex-matched non-stroke patients (control group) (Figure 14). The CCS was significantly higher in the stroke group than the control group (median 64 vs. 3, $p < 0.0001$). No calcium was found in 23.2% and 47.7% ($p < 0.001$), respectively. CCS >400 was detected in 24.5% and 9.3% ($p < 0.001$), respectively. Agreement between the FRS and CCS was found in only 62 patients (41.1%). In a multiple logistic regression analysis, age (HR 1.09/year, 95% CI 1.03—1.14, $p = 0.001$), diabetes (HR 2.97, 95% CI 1.52—5.78, $p = 0.001$), stroke (HR 3.85, 95% CI 1.89—7.81, $p = 0.001$), and male sex (HR 4.41, 95% CI 1.82—0.75, $p = 0.001$) were significantly associated with CCS >400. Thus, our results show that the prevalence of subclinical CAD in ischemic stroke patients was very high, and that a quarter had CCS >400. Age, diabetes, stroke, and male sex were independent predictors of high-risk CCS.

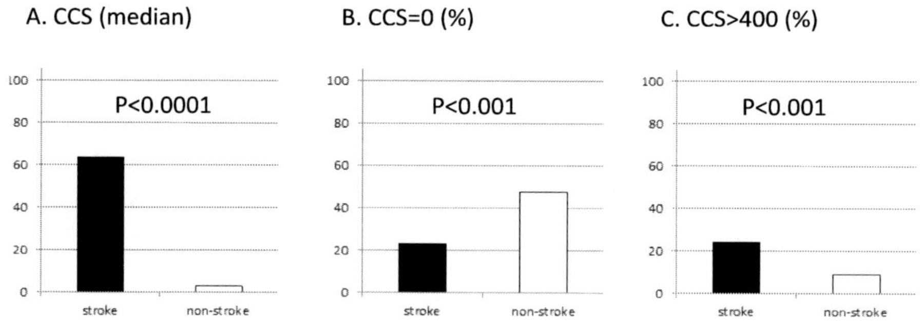

Figure 14. Stroke. A: Median value of coronary calcium score (CCS), B: Prevalence of CCS of 0, C: Prevalence of CCS >400. Modified from Iwasaki et al. [87].

Yoo et al. [88] performed CCTA in 1,304 stroke patients. They found that the frequency of significant stenosis was 32.3%. One study [89] evaluated 104 patients with cerebral infarction and found a prevalence of significant stenosis of 37.5%. Another study [90] performed CCTA in 274 patients with nondisabling, non-cardioembolic ischemic stroke or transient ischemic attack and no known CAD [63], and found significant stenosis in 18% of patients. Thus, previous studies have shown that 20-40% of stroke patients have asymptomatic significant stenosis.

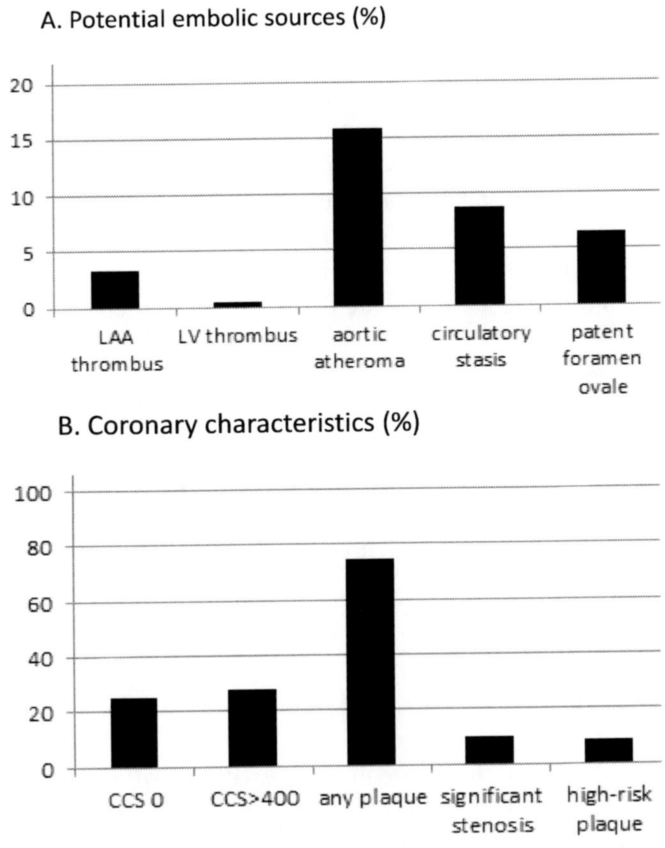

Figure 15. Embolic stroke. A: Potential embolic sources, B: Coronary characteristics. Modified from Iwasaki et al. [91].

Identification of Cardiac Embolic Sources

We performed MDCT in 184 patients with embolic stroke but without known CAD [91]. Twenty-six patients had atrial fibrillation. Overall, 64 potential embolic sources were detected in 59 patients (32.1%, Figure 15 A). As high-risk sources, left atrial appendage thrombus, left ventricular thrombus, and aortic atheroma were detected in 3.3%, 0.5%, and 15.8% of patients, respectively. As medium-risk sources, circulatory stasis and patent foramen ovale were detected in 8.7% and 6.5%, respectively. Coronary characteristics of these patients are shown in Figure 15 B. As for CCS, only 47 patients (25.5%) had zero CCS and 51 (27.7%) had CCS >400. A total of 137 patients (74.5%) had any coronary plaques. Significant stenosis was detected in 18 patients (9.8%). The prevalence of high-risk plaque was 8.7% (PR 7.1%, LAP 1.6%, spotty calcification 5.4%, and a napkin-ring sign 2.7%). Importantly, only 34 patients (13.0%) had no abnormalities detected by MDCT. Thus, our results suggest that MDCT has a potential to identify both cardiac embolic sources and CAD in patients with embolic stroke but without known CAD.

Previous studies investigated the prevalence of CAD in patients with ischemic stroke or transient ischemic attack (TIA) but without known CAD [88-90]. These studies have shown that 20-40% of stroke patients had asymptomatic significant CAD. However, these studies excluded patients with embolic stroke. Only a few reports studied patients with embolic stroke. One study [92] performed CCTA in 175 patients suspected to have had embolic stroke/TIA; atherosclerotic plaques were identified in 60%, and 21% had occult significant stenosis. Another study [93] found significant stenosis in 36% of 200 patients with ischemic stroke but without known atrial fibrillation or CAD. Our results showed that 75% of patients had any coronary plaques and 10% had significant stenosis. Surprisingly, 8 of 18 among our patients had a chronic total occlusion. Thus, subclinical atherosclerosis is highly prevalent in embolic stroke patients.

CCTA for the Evaluation of Statin Therapy

Statins are a mainstay in the treatment of patients with CAD. Many large trials of statin therapy demonstrated a 28% decrease in low-density lipoprotein-cholesterol (LDL-C), and a 5-year statin trial was associated with a 25% to 35% drop in CAD risk, leaving a substantial residual risk [94].

We [95] studied whether standard statin therapy would prevent progression of CAD and carotid artery disease in asymptomatic patients without known CAD. We retrospectively selected 45 patients who continued statin therapy for 1 year and underwent MDCT and carotid ultrasound measurement 1 year apart (Figure 16 and 17). The follow-up period was 1.37±0.49 years. Total cholesterol decreased from 213.2±46.2 mg/dl to 196.0±34.3 mg/dl ($p = 0.045$). Triglyceride decreased from 125.5±72.3 mg/dl to 107.1±58.2 mg/dl ($p = 0.184$). High-density lipoprotein (HDL)-cholesterol decreased from 60.8 ± 15.8 mg/dl to 60.0 ± 12.3 mg/dl ($p = 0.789$). LDL-cholesterol increased from 101.7 ± 25.2 mg/dl to 102.7±23.0 mg/dl (p = 0.844). However, CCS significantly increased (median 57 to 83, p = 0.009), and the mean number of coronary plaques significantly increased (2.5 ± 1.7 to 3.0 ± 1.7, p = 0.001). Carotid IMT also significantly increased (1.42 ± 0.81 to 1.78 ± 0.92, p = 0.049), and the mean number of carotid plaques significantly increased (0.5 ± 1.1 to 1.1 ± 1.5, p = 0.001). Thus, our results showed that CAD and carotid artery disease progressed significantly despite normal lipid values using standard statin therapy in asymptomatic patients without known CAD. This suggests that more intense lipid lowering will be needed to prevent progression of CAD and carotid artery disease.

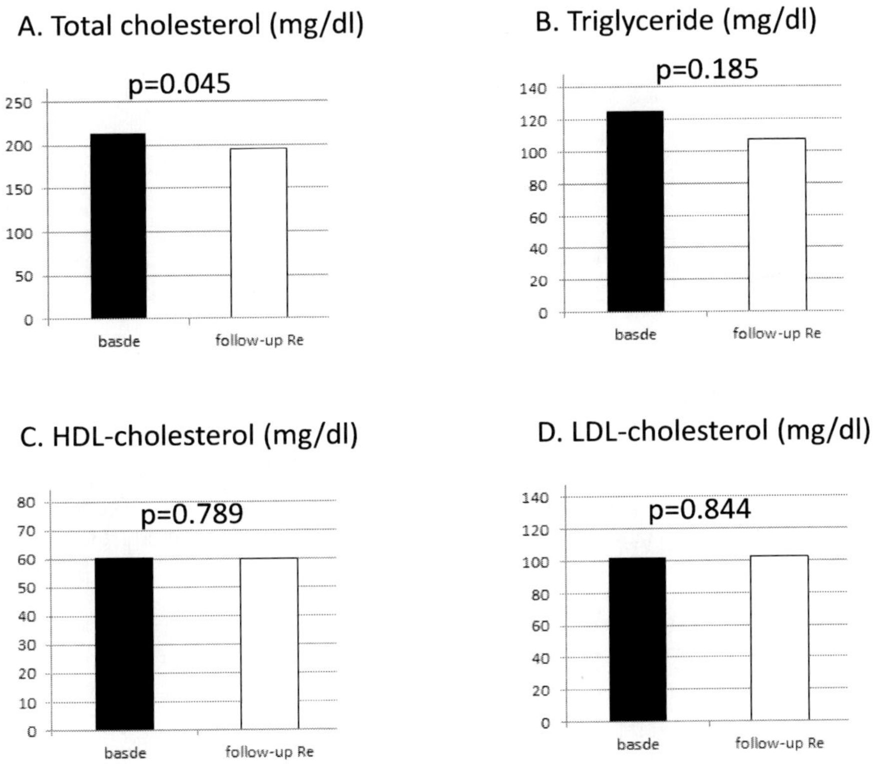

Figure 16. Statin therapy (changes of lipids). A: Change of total cholesterol, B: Change of triglyceride, C: Change of HDL-cholesterol, D: Change of LDL-cholesterol. Modified from Iwasaki et al. [95].

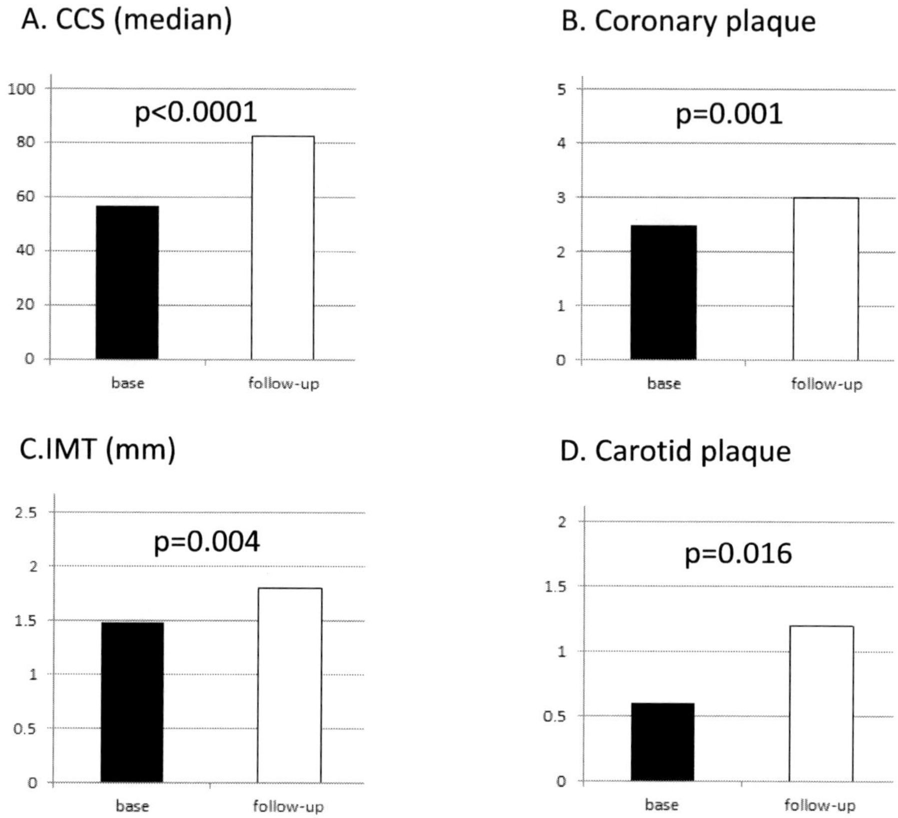

Figure 17. Statin therapy. A: Change of median value of coronary calcium score (CCS), B: Change of mean number of coronary plaques, C: Change of intima media thickness (IMT), D: Change of mean number of carotid plaques. Modified from Iwasaki et al. [95].

There are several therapeutic studies demonstrating the effects of statin therapy on CCS [96-98]. Most studies showed that statins reduced the progression rate of CCS compared with placebo. However, studies that compared intensive statin therapy with standard statin therapy showed no significant change in progression rate of CCS and no correlation of CCS with changes in LDL-C levels [99-102]. Thus, statins have been unsuccessful in reducing CAD progression. On the other hand, intravascular ultrasound studies have demonstrated that plaque regression is observed when LDL-C decreases below 70-80 mg/dl [103]. Thus, intensive lowering of LDL-C below 80 mg/dl will be needed to prevent the progression of CAD. Representative cases of plaque progression and regression are shown in Figure 18 and 19.

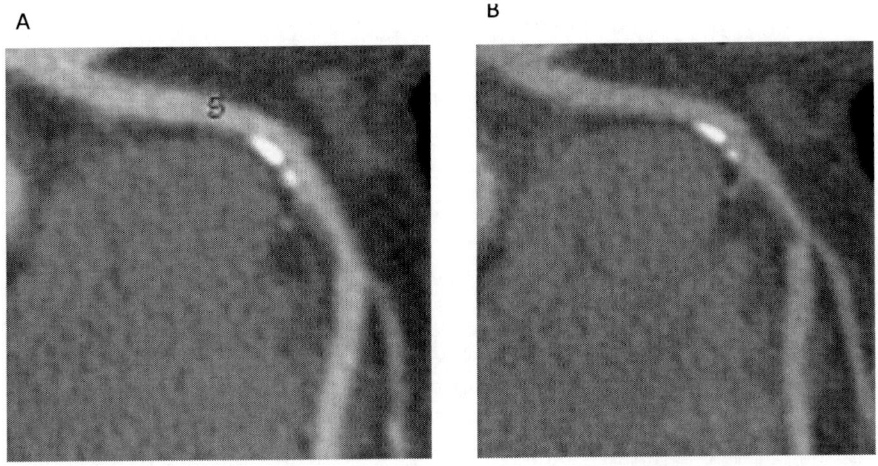

Figure 18. Plaque progression. Plaque progression was observed in a 64-years-old man despite one year of standard statin therapy. A. baseline, B. follow-up.

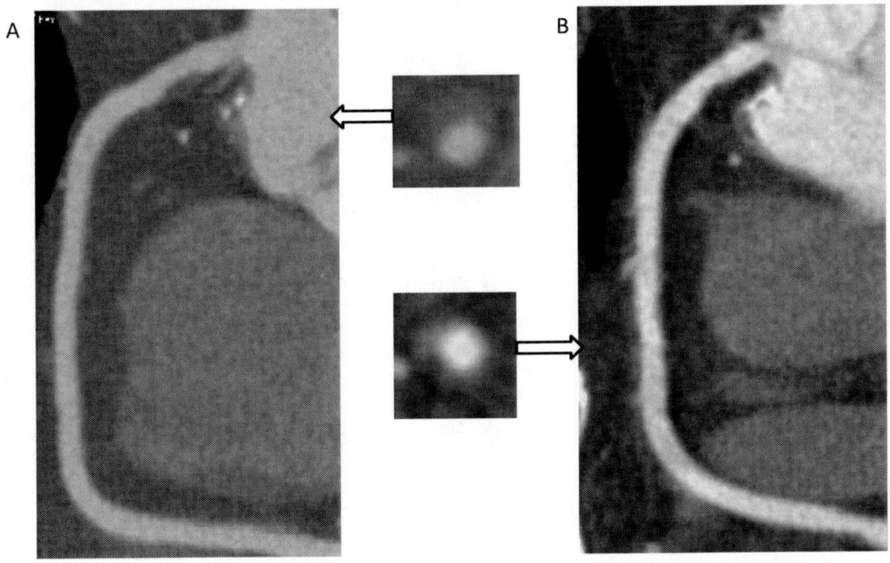

Figure 19. Plaque regression. Plaque regression was observed in a 68-years-old man after one year of high-intensity statin therapy. A. baseline, B. follow-up.

Radiation Safety and Contrast Media

Radiation doses associated with CCTA exceed those for invasive coronary angiography, and a typical effective dose is 8-30 mSv [104]. However, recent technical advances, such as tube current modulation, prospectively triggered axial acquisition, and prospectively electrocardiogram-triggered high-pitch spiral acquisition, reduced radiation dose to the 1 mSv range [105-108].

Safe and effective clinical use of contrast media is important in CCTA. Contrast-induced nephropathy (CIN) is usually defined as either an absolute change in serum creatinine of greater than 0.5 mg/dl or a greater than 25% increase in serum creatinine from baseline within 2 to 3 days following exposure to the contrast agent [109]. Risk factors associated with the development of CIN are hypotension, congestive heart failure, CKD, diabetes, elderly (>75 years old), anemia, and contrast volume [110]. Intravenous infusion of 0.9% saline has been the simplest and most effective measure to prevent contrast-induced nephropathy [111]. Moreover, recent technical advances have reduced the dose of contrast media from 70-100 ml to 40 ml [112, 113].

Clinical Perspective

Current clinical guidelines do not support an indication for MDCT in the evaluation of patients without known CAD. In the 2010 ACCF/AHA (American College of Cardiology Foundation/American Heart Association) Guideline for Assessment of Cardiovascular Risk in Asymptomatic Adults [114], CCTA is not recommended for cardiovascular risk assessment in asymptomatic adults (Class III: No Benefit, Level of Evidence: C). For CCS, it is Class IIa (Level of Evidence: B) for asymptomatic adults at intermediate risk (10% to 20% 10-year risk). It is Class IIb (Level of Evidence: B) and Class III (Level of Evidence: B) for asymptomatic adults at low to intermediate risk (6% to 10% 10-year risk) and those at low risk (<6% 10-year risk), respectively. In the ACCF/ACR/AHA/NASCI/SAIP/PCAI/SCCT 2010 Expert Consensus Document on Coronary Computed Tomographic Angiography [115], non-calcified coronary plaque imaging is considered of uncertain clinical utility and is limited to research uses. Use of CCTA in asymptomatic high-risk individuals is considered an area without consensus. However, our results and some recent studies suggest that subclinical CAD in patients with low to intermediate risk is highly prevalent. Thus, MDCT may be considered as a useful modality to detect subclinical CAD in these populations.

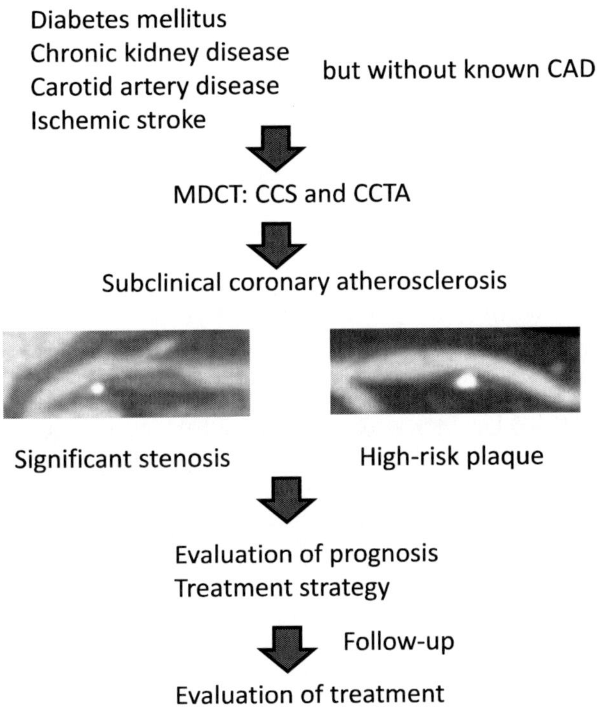

Figure 20. Role of multi-detector computed tomography in the management of patients without known coronary artery disease. Abbreviations: CAD, coronary artery disease; CCS, coronary calcium score; CCTA, coronary computed tomographic angiography; MDCT, multi-detector computed tomography.

In summary, these studies suggest that MDCT can detect subclinical coronary atherosclerosis in asymptomatic patients without known CAD, and has potential utility as the first study to evaluate patients with coronary risk factors but without known CAD (Figure 20). Subclinical coronary atherosclerosis in patients with low to intermediate risk but without known CAD is highly prevalent. Also, the prevalence of high-risk CAD is high in patients with diabetes, stroke, CKD, and carotid artery disease but without known CAD.

ACKNOWLEDGMENTS

I wish to thank Dr. Shozo Kusachi, Professor Emeritus at Okayama University, for providing critical comments and review of the manuscript. I also wish to thank Mr. Takeshi Matsumoto, R. T. for his technical support of MDCT procedure.

Conflict of Interest

None.

REFERENCES

[1] Roth GA, Huffman MD, Moran AE, Feigin V, Mensah GA, Naghavi M, Murray CJ. Global and Regional Patterns in Cardiovascular Mortality From 1990 to 2013. *Circulation.* 2015; 132: 1667-78.

[2] Schatzkin A, Cupples LA, Heeren T, Morelock S, Kannel WB. Sudden death in the Framingham Heart Study, Differences in incidence and risk factors by sex and coronary disease status. *Am J Epidemiol* 1984; 120: 888-99.

[3] Gibbons RJ, Jones DW, Gardner TJ, Goldstein LB, Moller JH, Yancy CW. The American Heart Association's 2008 statement of principles for healthcare reform. *Circulation* 2008; 118: 2209-18.

[4] Catapano AL, Reiner Z, De Backer G, Graham I, Taskinen MR, Wiklund O, Agewall S, Alegria E, Chapman M, Durrington P, Erdine S, Halcox J, Hobbs R, Kjekshus J, Filardi PP, Riccardi G, Storey RF, Wood D; European Society of Cardiology (ESC); European Atherosclerosis Society (EAS). ESC/EAS Guidelines for the management of dyslipidaemias The Task Force for the management of dyslipidaemias of the European Society of Cardiology (ESC) and the European Atherosclerosis Society (EAS). *Atherosclerosis.* 2011; 217: 3-46.

[5] Wang TJ. Assessing the role of circulating, genetic, and imaging biomarkers in cardiovascular risk prediction. *Circulation.* 2011; 123: 551-65.

[6] Ylä-Herttuala S, Bentzon JF, Daemen M, Falk E, Garcia-Garcia HM, Herrmann J, Hoefer I, Jauhiainen S, Jukema JW, Krams R, Kwak BR, Marx N, Naruszewicz M, Newby A, Pasterkamp G, Serruys PW, Waltenberger J, Weber C, Tokgözoglu L; ESC Working Group of Atherosclerosis and Vascular Biology. Stabilization of atherosclerotic plaques: an update. *Eur Heart J* 2013; 34: 3251-8.

[7] Perk J, De Backer G, Gohlke H, Graham I, Reiner Z, Verschuren M, Albus C, Benlian P, Boysen G, Cifkova R, Deaton C, Ebrahim S, Fisher M, Germano G, Hobbs R, Hoes A, Karadeniz S, Mezzani A, Prescott E, Ryden L, Scherer M, Syvänne M, Scholte op Reimer WJ, Vrints C, Wood D, Zamorano JL, Zannad F; European Association for Cardiovascular Prevention & Rehabilitation (EACPR); ESC Committee for Practice Guidelines (CPG). European Guidelines on cardiovascular disease prevention in clinical practice (version 2012). The Fifth Joint Task Force of the European Society of Cardiology and Other Societies on Cardiovascular Disease Prevention in Clinical Practice (constituted by representatives of nine societies and by invited experts). *Eur Heart J* 2012; 33: 1635-701.

[8] Shaw LJ, Taylor A, Raggi P, Berman DS. Role of noninvasive imaging in asymptomatic high-risk patients. *J Nucl Cardiol* 2006; 13: 156-62.

[9] Erbel R, Budoff M. Improvement of cardiovascular risk prediction using coronary imaging: subclinical atherosclerosis: the memory of lifetime risk factor exposure. *Eur Heart J* 2012; 33: 1201-13.

[10] Agatston AS, Janowitz WR, Hildner FJ, Zusmer NR, Viamonte M Jr., Detrano R. Quantification of coronary artery calcium using ultrafast computed tomography. *J Am Coll Cardiol* 1990; 15: 827-32.

[11] Rumberger JA, Simons DB, Fitzpatrick LA, Sheedy PF, Schwartz RS. Coronary artery calcium area by electron-beam computed tomography and coronary atherosclerotic plaque area. A histopathologic correlative study. *Circulation* 1995; 92: 2157-62.

[12] Sangiorgi G, Rumberger JA, Severson A, Edwards WD, Gregorie J, Fitzpatrick LA, Schwartz RS. Arterial calcification and not lumen stenosis is highly correlated with atherosclerotic plaque burden in humans: a histologic study of 723 coronary artery segments using nondecdalcifying methodology. *J Am Coll Cardiol* 1998; 31: 126-33.

[13] Baumgart D, Schmermund A, Görge G, Haude M, Ge J, Adamzik M, Sehnert C, Altmaier K, Grönemeyer D, Seibel R, Erbel R. Comparison of electron-beam computed tomography with intracoronary ultrasound

and coronary angiography for detection of coronary atherosclerosis. *J Am Coll Cardiol* 1997; 30: 57-64.

[14] Schmermund A, Baumgart D, Görge G, Seibel R, Grönemeyer D, Ge J, Haude M, Rumberger J, Erbel R. Coronary artery calcium in acute coronary syndrome: a comparative study of electron-beam computed tomography, coronary angiography, and intracoronary ultrasound in survivors of acute myocardial infarction and unstable angina. *Circulation* 1997; 96: 1461-9.

[15] Arad Y, Spadaro LA, Goodman K, Newstein D, Guerci AD. Prediction of coronary events with electron beam computed tomography. *J Am Coll Cardiol* 2000; 36: 1253-60.

[16] Kondos GT, Hoff JA, Sevrukov A, Daviglus ML, Garside DS, Devries SS, Chomka EV, Liu K. Electron-beam tomography coronary artery calcium and cardiac events: a 37-months follow-up of 5635 initially asymptom atic low- to intermediate-risk adults. *Circulation* 2003; 107: 2571-6.

[17] Raggi P, Callister TQ, Cooil B, He ZX, Lippolis NJ, Russo DJ, Zelinger A, Mahmarian JJ. Identification of patients at increased risk of first unheralded acute myocardial infarction by electron-beam computed tomography. *Circulation* 2000; 101: 850-5.

[18] Kondos GT, Hoff JA, Sevrukov A, Daviglus ML, Garside DB, Devries SS, Chomka EV, Liu K. Electron-beam tomography coronary artery calcium and cardiac events: a 37-months follow-up of 5635 initially asymptomatic low- to intermediate-risk adults. *Circulation* 2003; 107: 2571-6.

[19] Greenland P, LaBree L, Azen SP, Doherty TM, Detrano RC. Coronary artery calcium score combined with Framingham score for risk prediction in asymptomatic individuals. *JAMA* 2004; 291: 210-5.

[20] Arad Y, Goodman KJ, Roth M, Newstein D, Guerci AD. Coronary calcification, coronary disease risk factors, C-reactive protein, and atherosclerotic cardiovascular disease events: the St. Francis Heart Study. *J Am Coll Cardiol* 2005; 46: 158-65.

[21] Abdulla J, Abildstrom SZ, Gotzsche O, Christensen E, Kober L, Torp-Pedersen C. 64-Multisclice detector computed tomography coronary angiography as potential alternative to conventional coronary angiography: a systematic review and meta-analysis. *Eur Heart J* 2007; 28: 3042-50.

[22] Hamon M, Biondi-Zoccai GG, Malagutti P, Agostoni P, Morello R, ValgimigliM, Hamon M. Diagnostic performance of multislice spiral

computed tomography of coronary arteries as compared with conventional invasive coronary angiography: a meta-analysis. *J Am Coll Cardiol* 2006; 48: 1896-910.

[23] Hamon M, Morello R, Riddle JW, Hamon M. Coronary arteries: diagnostic performance of 16- versus 64-section spiral CT compared with invasive coronary angiography- meta-analysis. *Radiology* 2007; 245: 720-31.

[24] Mowatt G, Cook JA, Hillis GS, Walker S, Fraser C, Jia X, Waugh N. 64-slice computed tomography angiography in the diagnosis and assessment of coronary artery disease; systemic review and meta-analysis. *Heart* 2008; 94: 1386-93.

[25] Miller JM, Rochitte CE, Dewey M, Arbab-Zadeh A, Niinuma H, Gottlieb I, Paul N, Clouse ME, Shapiro EP, Hoe J, Lardo AC, Bush DE, de Roos A, Cox C, Brinker J, Lima JA. Diagnostic performance of coronary angiography by 64-row CT. *N Engl J Med* 2008; 359: 2324-36.

[26] Budoff MJ, Dowe D, Jollis JG, Gitter M, Sutherland J, Halamert E, Scherer M, Bellinger R, Martin A, Benton R, Delago A, Min JK. Diagnostic performance of 64-multidetector row coronary computed tomographic angiography for evaluation of coronary artery stenosis in individuals without known coronary artery disease: results from the prospective multicenter ACCURACY (Assessment by Coronary Computed Tomographic Angiography of Individuals Undergoing Invasive Coronary Angiography) trial. *J Am Coll Cardiol* 2008; 52: 1724-32.

[27] Meijboom WB, Meijs MF, Schuijf JD, Cramer MJ, Mollet NR, van Mieghem CA, Nieman K, van Werkhoven JM, Pundziute G, Weustink AC, de Vos AM, Pugliese F, Rensing B, Jukema JW, Bax JJ, Prokop M, Doevendans PA, Hunink MG, Krestin GP, de Feyter PJ. Diagnostic accuracy of 64-slice computed tomography coronary angiography: a prospective, multicenter, multivendor study. *J Am Coll Cardiol* 2008; 52: 2135-44.

[28] Achenbach S, Moselewski F, Ropers D, Ferencik M, Hoffmann U, MacNeill B, Pohle K, Baum U, Anders K, Jang IK, Daniel WG, Brady TJ. Detection of calcified and noncalcified coronary atherosclerotic plaque by contrast-enhanced, submillimeter multidetector spiral computed tomography. A segment-based comparison with intravascular ultrasound. *Circulation* 2004; 109: 14-17.

[29] Leber AW, Knez A, Becker A, Becker C, von Zieger F, Nikolaou K, Rist C, Reiser M, White C, Steinbeck G, Boekstegers P. Accuracy of

multidetector spiral computed tomography in identifying and differentiating the composition of coronary atherosclerotic plaques: a comparative study with intravascular ultrasound. *J Am Coll Cardiol* 2004; 43: 1241-7.

[30] Leber AW, Knez A, von Zieger F, Becker A, Nikolaou K, Paul S, Wintersperger B, Reiser M, Becker CR, Steinbeck G, Boekstegers P. Quantitation of obstructive and nonobstructive coronary lesions by 64-slice computed tomography. A comparative study withquantitative coronary angiography and intravascular ultrasound. *J Am Coll Cardiol* 2005; 46: 147-54.

[31] Leber AW, Becker A, Knez A, von Zieger F, Sirol M, Nikolaou K, Ohnesorge B, Fayad ZA, Becker CR, Reiser M, Steinbeck G, Boekstegers P. Accuracy of 64-slice computed tomography to classify and quantify plaque volumes in the proximal coronary system. *J Am Coll Cardiol* 2006; 47: 672-7.

[32] Ferencik M, Nieman K, Achenbach S. Noncalcified and calcified coronary plaque detection by contrast-enhanced multi-detector computed tomography: a study of interobserver agreement. *J Am Coll Cardiol* 2006; 47: 207-209.

[33] Min JK, Dunning A, Lin FY, Achenbach S, Al-Mallah M, Budoff MJ, Cademartiri F, Callister TQ, Chang HJ, Cheng V, Chinnaiyan K, Chow BJ, Delago A, Hadamitzky M, Hausleiter J, Kaufmann P, Maffei E, Raff G, Shaw LJ, Villines T, Berman DS; CONFIRM Investigators. Age- and sex-related differences in all-cause mortality risk based on coronary computed tomography angiography findings results from the International Multicenter CONFIRM (Coronary CT Angiography Evaluation for Clinical Outcomes: An International Multicenter Registry) of 23,854 patients without known coronary artery disease. J *Am Coll Cardiol* 2011; 58: 849-60.

[34] Hou ZH, Lu B, Gao Y, Jiang SL, Wang Y, Li W, Budoff MJ. Prognostic value of coronary CT angiography and calcium score for major adverse cardiac events in outpatients. *JACC Cardiovasc Imaging* 2012; 5: 990-99.

[35] Arbab-Zadeh A, Nakano M, Virmani R, Fuste V. Acute coronary events. *Circulation* 2012; 125:1147-56.

[36] Libby P. Mechanism of acute coronary syndromes and their implacations for therapy. *N Engl J Med* 2013; 368: 2004-13.

[37] Bamberg F, Sommer WH, Hoffmann V, Achenbach S, Nikolaou K, Conen D, Reiser MF, Hoffmann U, Becker CR. Meta-analysis and

systematic review of the long-term predictive value of assessment of coronary atherosclerosis by contrast-enhanced coronary computed tomography angiography. *J Am Coll Cardiol* 2011; 57: 2426-36.

[38] Hulten EA, Carbonaro S, Petrillo SP, Mitchell JD, Villines TC. Prognostic value of cardiac computed tomography angiography: a systematic review and meta-analysis. *J Am Coll Cardiol* 2011; 57: 1237-47.

[39] Motoyama S, Kondo T, Sarai M, Sugiura A, Harigaya H, Sato T, Inoue K, Okumura M, Ishii J, Anno H, Virmani R, Ozaki Y, Hishida H, Narula J. Multislice computed tomographic characteristics of coronary lesions in acute coronary syndromes. *J Am Coll Cardiol* 2007; 50: 319-26.

[40] Otsuka K, Fukuda S, Tanaka A, Nakanishi K, Taguchi H, Yoshikawa J, Shimada K, Yoshiyama M. Napkin-ring sign on coronary CT angiography for the prediction of acute coronary syndrome. *JACC Cardiovasc Imaging* 2013; 6: 448-57.

[41] Motoyama S, Sarai M, Harigaya H, Anno H, Inoue K, Hara T, Naruse H, Ishii J, Hishida H, Wong ND, Virmani R, Kondo T, Ozaki Y, Narula J. Computed tomographic angiography characteristics of atherosclerotic plaques subsequently resulting in acute coronary syndrome. *J Am Coll Cardiol* 2009; 54: 49-57.

[42] Fernández-Friera L, Peñalvo JL, Fernández-Ortiz A, Ibañez B, López-Melgar B, Laclaustra M, Oliva B, Mocoroa A, Mendiguren J, Martínez de Vega V, García L, Molina J, Sánchez-González J, Guzmán G, Alonso-Farto JC, Guallar E, Civeira F, Sillesen H, Pocock S, Ordovás JM, Sanz G, Jiménez-Borreguero LJ, Fuster V. Prevalence, Vascular Distribution, and Multiterritorial Extent of Subclinical Atherosclerosis in a Middle-Aged Cohort: The PESA (Progression of Early Subclinical Atherosclerosis) Study. *Circulation* 2015; 131: 2104-13.

[43] Sillesen H, Muntendam P, Adourian A, Entrekin R, Garcia M, Falk E, Fuster V. Carotid plaque burden as a measure of subclinical atherosclerosis: comparison with other tests for subclinical arterial disease in the High Risk Plaque BioImage study. *JACC Cardiovasc Imaging* 2012; 5: 681-9.

[44] Baber U, Mehran R, Sartori S, Schoos MM, Sillesen H, Muntendam P, Garcia MJ, Gregson J, Pocock S, Falk E, Fuster V. Prevalence, impact, and predictive value of detecting subclinical coronary and carotid atherosclerosis in asymptomatic adults: the BioImage study. *J Am Coll Cardiol* 2015; 65: 1065-74.

[45] Iwasaki K, Matsumoto T, Aono H, Furukawa H, Samukawa M. Prevalence of subclinical atherosclerosis in asymptomatic patients with low to intermediate risk by 64-slice computed tomography. *Coron Artery Dis* 2011; 22:18-25.

[46] NIPPON DATA80 Research Group. Risk assessment chart for death from cardiovascular disease based on a 19-year follow-up study of a Japanese representative population. *Circ J* 2006; 70: 1249-55.

[47] Hausleiter J, Meyer T, Hadamitzky M, Kastrati A, Martinoff S, Schömig A. Prevalence of noncalcified coronary plaques by 64-slice computed tomography in patients with an intermediate risk for significant coronary artery disease. *J Am Coll Cardiol* 2006; 48: 312-18.

[48] Choi EK, Choi SI, Rivera JJ, Nasir K, Chang SA, Chun EJ, Kim HK, Choi DJ, Blumenthal RS, Chang HJ. Coronary computed tomography angiography as a screening tool for the detection of occult coronary artery disease in asymptomatic individuals. *J Am Coll Cardiol* 2008; 52: 357-65.

[49] Iwasaki K, Matsumoto T, Aono H, Furukawa H, Samukawa M. Prevalence of non-calcified coronary plaque on 64-slice computed tomography in asymptomatic patients with zero and low coronary artery calcium. *Can J Cardiol* 2010; 26: 377-80.

[50] Cheng VY, Lepor NE, Madyoon H, Fshaghian S, Naraghi AL, Shah PK. Presence and severity of noncalcified coronary plaque on 64-slice computed tomographic coronary angiography in patients with zero and low coronary artery calcium. *Am J Cardiol* 2007; 99: 1183-6.

[51] Schroeder S, Kuettner A, Kopp AF, Heuschmidt M, Burgstahler C, Herdeg C, Claussen CD. Noninvasive evaluation of the prevalence of noncalcified atherosclerotic plaques by multi-slice detector computed tomography: results of a pilot study. *Int J Cardiol* 2003; 92: 151-5.

[52] Rubinshtein R, Gasper T, Halon DA, Goldstein J, Peled N, Lewis BS. Prevalence and extent of obstructive coronary artery disease in patients with zero or low calcium score undergoing 64-slice cardiac multidetector computed tomography for evaluation of a chest pain syndrome. *Am J Cardiol* 2007; 99: 472-5.

[53] Iwasaki K, Matsumoto T, Aono H, Furukawa H, Nagamachi K, Samukawa M. Distribution of coronary atherosclerosis in patients with coronary artery disease. *Heart Vessels* 2010; 25: 14-8.

[54] Halon DA, Sapoznikov D, Lewis BS, Gotsman MS. Localization of lesions in the coronary circulation. *Am J Cardiol* 1983; 52: 921-6.

[55] Tuzcu EM, Kapadia SR, Tutar E, Ziada KM, Hobbs RE, McCarthy PM, Young JB, Nissen SE. High prevalence of coronary atherosclerosis in asymptomatic teenagers and young adults: evidence from intravascular ultrasound. *Circulation* 2001; 103: 2705-10.

[56] Schmermund A, Baumgart D, Möhlenkamp S, Kriener P, Pump H, Grönemeyer D, Seibel R, Erbel R. Natural history and topographic pattern of progression of coronary calcification in symptomatic patients: An electron-beam CT study. *Arterioscler Thromb Vasc Biol* 2001; 21: 421-6.

[57] Mazurek T, Zhang L, Zalewski A, Mannion JD, Diehl JT, Arafat H, Sarov-Blat L, O'Brien S, Keiper EA, Johnson AG, Martin J, Goldstein BJ, Shi Y. Human epicardial adipose tissue is a source of inflammatory mediators. *Circulation* 2003; 108: 2460-6.

[58] Iacobellis G, Pistilli D, Gucciardo M, Leonetti F, Miraldi F, Brancaccio G, Gallo P, di Gioia CR. Adiponectin expression in human epicardial adipose tissue in vivo is lower in patients with coronary artery disease. *Cytokine* 2005; 21: 251-5.

[59] Baker AR, Silva NF, Quinn DW, Harte AL, Pagano D, Bonser RS, Kumar S, McTernan PG. Human epicardial adipose tissue expresses a pathogenic profile of adipocytokines in patients with cardiovascular disease. *Cardiovasc Diabetol* 2006; 5: 1.

[60] Iwasaki K, Matsumoto T, Aono H, Furukawa H, Samukawa M. Relationship between epicardial fat measured by 64-multidetector computed tomography and coronary artery disease. *Clin Cardiol* 2011; 34: 166-71.

[61] Gorter PM, de Vos AM, van der Graaf Y, Stella PR, Doevendans PA, Meijs MF, Prokop M, Visseren FL. Relation of epicardial and pericoronary fat to coronary atherosclerosis and coronary artery calcium in patients undergoing coronary angiography. *Am J Cardiol* 2008; 102: 380-5.

[62] Djaberi R, Schuijf JD, van Werkhoven JM, Nucifora G, Jukema JW, Bax JJ. Relation of epicardial adipose tissue to coronary atherosclerosis. *Am J Cardiol* 2008; 102: 1602-7.

[63] Ueno K, Anzai T, Jinzaki M, Yamada M, Jo Y, Maekawa Y, Kawamura A, Yoshikawa T, Tanami Y, Sato K, Kuribayashi S, Ogawa S. Increased epicardial fat volume quantified by 64-multidetector computed tomography is associated with coronary athrosclerosis and totally occlusive lesions. *Circ J* 2009: 73: 1927-33.

[64] Redberg RF, Greenland P, Fuster V, Pyörälä K, Blair SN, Folsom AR, Newman AB, O'Leary DH, Orchard TJ, Psaty B, Schwartz JS, Starke R, Wilson PW. Prevention Conference VI: Diabetes and Cardiovascular Disease: Writing Group III: risk assessment in persons with diabetes. *Circulation* 2002; 105: e144-52.

[65] Haffner SM, Lehto S, Rönnemaa T, Pyörälä K, Laakso M. Mortality from coronary heart disease in subjects with type 2 diabetes and in nondiabetic subjects with and without prior myocardial infarction. *N Engl J Med* 1998; 339: 229-34.

[66] Libby P, Nathan DM, Abraham K, Brunzell JD, Fradkin JE, Haffner SM, Hsueh W, Rewers M, Roberts BT, Savage PJ, Skarlatos S, Wassef M, Rabadan-Diehl C; National Heart, Lung, and Blood Institute; National Institute of Diabetes and Digestive and Kidney Diseases Working Group on Cardiovascular Complications of Type 1 Diabetes Mellitus. Report of the National Heart, Lung, and Blood Institute-National Institute of Diabetes and Digestive and Kidney Diseases Working Group on Cardiovascular Complications of Type 1 Diabetes Mellitus. *Circulation* 2005; 111: 3489-93.

[67] Iwasaki K, Matsumoto T, Aono H, Furukawa H, Samukawa M. Prevalence of subclinical atherosclerosis in asymptomatic diabetic patients by 64-slice computed tomography. *Coron Artery Dis* 2008; 19: 195-202.

[68] Khaleeli E, Peters SR, Bobrowsky K, Oudiz RJ, Ko JY, Budoff MJ. Diabetes and the associated incidence of subclinical atherosclerosis and coronary artery disease: Implication for management. *Am Heart J* 2001; 141: 637-44.

[69] Pundziute G, Schuijf JD, Jukema JW, Boersma E, Scholte AJ, Kroft LJ, van der Wall EE, Bax JJ. Noninvasive assessment of plaque characteristics with multislice computed tomography coronary angiography in symptomatic diabetic patients. *Diabetes Care* 2007; 30: 1113-9.

[70] Maffei E, Seitun S, Nieman K, Martini C, Guaricci AI, Tedeschi C, Weustink AC, Mollet NR, Berti E, Grilli R, Messalli G, Cademartiri F. Assessment of coronary artery disease and calcified coronary plaque burden by computed tomography in patients with and without diabetes mellitus. *Eur Radiol* 2011; 21: 944-53.

[71] Iwasaki K, Matsumoto T. Characteristics of subclinical coronary artery disease in diabetic patients without known coronary artery disease. *Journal of Research in Diabetes* Vol. 2014 (2014), Article ID 322292

[72] Iwasaki K, Matsumoto T, Hasegawa K. Predictors of high-risk coronary artery disease detected by coronary computed tomographic angiography in diabetic patients without known coronary artery disease. *Int J Cardiol* 2015; 201: 324-5.

[73] Kim JJ, Hwang BH, Choi IJ, Choo EH, Lim S, Kim JK, Koh YS, Kim DB, Jang SW, Cho EJ, Lee JM, Kim PJ, Cho JH, Jung JI, Seung KB, Min JK, Chang K. Impact of diabetes duration on the extent and severity of coronary atheroma burden and long-term clinical outcome in asymptomatic type 2 diabetic patients: evaluation by Coronary CT angiography. *Eur Heart J Cardiovasc Imaging* 2015; 16: 1065-73.

[74] Mitsutake R, Miura S, Shiga Y, Kawamura A, Saku K. Is chronic kidney disease associated with coronary artery stenosis or calcification as assessed by multi-detector row computed tomography? *Intern Med* 2008; 47: 1835-41.

[75] Cho I, Min HS, Chun EJ, Park SK, Choi Y, Blumenthal RS, Rivera JJ, Nasir K, Kim YJ, Sohn DW, Oh BH, Park YB, Chang HJ. Coronary atherosclerosis detected by coronary CT angiography in asymptomatic subjects with early chronic kidney disease. *Atherosclerosis* 2010; 208:406-11.

[76] Kawai H, Sarai M, Motoyama S, Harigaya H, Ito H, Sanda Y, Biswas S, Anno H, Ishii J, Murohara T, Ozaki Y. Coronary plaque characteristics in patients with mild chronic kidney disease. Analysis by 320-row area detector computed tomography. *Circ J* 2012; 76: 1436-41.

[77] Iwasaki K, Matsumoto T, Furukawa H, Samukawa M. Prevalence of coronary artery disease in asymptomatic patients with abnormal intima-media thickness by 64-slice computed tomography. *Int J Cardiol* 2010; 144: 119-20.

[78] Pignoli P, Tremoli E, Poli A, Oreste P, Paoletti R. Intimal plus medial thickness of the arterial wall: a direct measurement with ultrasound imaging. *Circulation* 1986; 74: 1399-406.

[79] Michell JR, Schwartz CJ. Relationship between arterial disease in different sites. A study of the aorta and coronary, carotid , and iliac arteries. *Br Med J* 1962; 1: 1293-301.

[80] Kullo IJ, Malik AR. Arterial ultrasonography and tonometry as a adjuncts to cardiovascular risk stratification. *J Am Coll Cardiol* 2007; 49: 1413-26.

[81] Bots ML, Hoes AW, Koudstaal PJ, Hofman A, Grobbee DE. Common carotid intima-media thickness nd risk of stroke and myocardial infarction: the Rotterdam Study. *Circulation* 1997; 96: 1432-1437.

[82] Hoeg JM. Evaluating coronary heart disease risk. Tiles in the mosaic. *JAMA* 1997; 277: 1387-1390.

[83] Hodis HN, Mack WJ, LaBree L, Selzer RH, Liu CR, Liu CH, Azen SP. The role of carotid arterial intima-media thickness in predicting clinical coronary events. *Ann Intern Med* 1998; 128: 262-269.

[84] Lorenz MW, Markus HS, Bots ML, Rosvall M, Sitzer M. Prediction of clinical cardiovascular events with carotid intima-media thickness. A systematic review and meta-analysis. *Circulation* 2007; 115: 459-467.

[85] Newman AB, Naydeck BL, Sutton-Tyrrell K, Edmundowicz D, O'Leary D, Kronmal R, Burke GL, Kuller LH. Relationship between coronary artery calcification and other measures of subclinical cardiovascular disease in older adults. *Arterioscler Thromb Vasc Biol* 2002; 22: 1674-1679.

[86] Lackland DT, Elkind MS, D'Agostino R Sr, Dhamoon MS, Goff DC Jr, Higashida RT, McClure LA, Mitchell PH, Sacco RL, Sila CA, Smith SC Jr, Tanne D, Tirschwell DL, Touzé E, Wechsler LR; on behalf of the American Heart Association Stroke Council, Council on Epidemiology and Prevention, Council on Cardiovascular Radiology and Intervention, Council on Cardiovascular Nursing, Council on Peripheral Vascular Disease, and Council on Quality of Care and Outcomes Research. Inclusion of Stroke in Cardiovascular Risk Prediction Instruments: A Statement for Healthcare Professionals From the American Heart Association/American Stroke Association. *Stroke* 2012; 43: 1998-2027.

[87] Iwasaki K, Haraoka K, Hamaguchi T, Imamura T, Kawada S, Ohno M, Kashihara K. Prevalence of subclinical coronary artery disease in ischemic stroke patients. *J Cardiol* 2015; 65: 71-75.

[88] Yoo J, Yang JH, Choi BW, Kim YD, Nam HS, Choi HY, Lee HS, Cha MJ, Choi D, Nam CM, Jang Y, Lee DH, Kim J, Heo JH. The frequency and risk of preclinical coronary artery disease detected using multichannel cardiac computed tomography in patients with ischemic stroke. *Cerebrovasc Dis* 2012; 33: 286-94.

[89] Hoshino A, Nakamura T, Enomoto S, Kawahito H, Kurata H, Nakahara Y, Ijichi T. Prevalence of coronary artery disease in Japanese patients with cerebral infarction. *Circ J* 2008; 72: 404-8.

[90] Calvet D, Touze E, Varenne O, Sablayrolles JL, Weber S, Mas JL. Prevalence of asymptomatic coronary artery disease in ischemic stroke patients. The PRECORIS study. *Circulation* 2010; 121: 1623-29.

[91] Iwasaki K, Matsumoto T, Kawada S. Potential utility of multidetector computed tomography to identify both cardiac embolic sources and

coronary artery disease in patients with embolic stroke. *Cardiology* 2016; 133: 205-10.

[92] Yoon YE, Chang HJ, Cho I, Jeon KH, Chun EJ, Choi SI, Bae HJ, Rivera JJ, Nasir K, Blumenthal RS, Lim TH: Incidence of subclinical coronary atherosclerosis in patients with suspected embolic stroke using cardiac computed tomography. *Int J Cardiovasc Imaging* 2011: 27: 1035-44.

[93] Kim SJ, Choe YH, Park SJ, Kim GM, Chung CS, Lee KH, Bang OY: Routine cardiac evaluation in patients with ischaemic stroke and absence of known atrial fibrillation or coronary heart disease: transthoracic echocardiography vs. multidetector cardiac computed tomography. *Eur J Neurol* 2012; 19: 317-23.

[94] O'Keefe JH Jr, Cordain L, Harris WH, Moe RM, Vogel R. Optimal low-density lipoprotein is 50 to 70 mg/dl: lower is better and physiologically normal. *J Am Coll Cardiol* 2004; 43: 2142-6.

[95] Iwasaki K, Matsumoto T. Coronary artery disease and carotid artery disease progress despite normal lipid levels by standard statin therapy in asymptomatic patients without known coronary artery disease: Implications for statin therapy. *Enliven: Clinical Cardiology and Research* 2014; 1;1-5.

[96] Callister TQ, Raggi P, Cooil B, Lippolis NJ, Russo DJ. Effect of HMG-CoA reductase inhibitors on coronary artery disease as assessed by electron-beam computed tomography. *N Engl J Med* 1998; 339: 1972-8.

[97] Achenbach S, Ropers D, Pohle K, Leber A, Thilo C, Knez A, Menendez T, Maeffert R, Kusus M, Regenfus M, Bickel A, Haberl R, Steinbeck G, Moshage W, Daniel WG. Influence of lipid-lowering therapy on the progression of coronary artery calcification: a prospective evaluation. *Circulation* 2002; 106: 1077-82.

[98] Raggi P, Davidson M, Callister TQ, Welty FK, Bachmann GA, Hecht H, Rumberger JA. Aggressive versus moderate lipid-lowering therapy in hypercholesterolemic postmenopausal women: Beyond Endorsed Lipid Lowering with EBT Scanning (BELLES). *Circulation* 2005; 112: 563-71.

[99] Schmermund A, Achenbach S, Budde T, Buziashvili Y, Förster A, Friedrich G, Henein M, Kerkhoff G, Knollmann F, Kukharchuk V, Lahiri A, Leischik R, Moshage W, Schartl M, Siffert W, Steinhagen-Thiessen E, Sinitsyn V, Vogt A, Wiedeking B, Erbel R. Effect of intensive versus standard lipid-lowering treatment with atorvastatin on the progression of calcified coronary atherosclerosis over 12 months: a

multicenter, randomized, double-blind trial. *Circulation* 2006; 113: 427-37.

[100] Houslay ES, Cowell SJ, Prescott RJ, Reid J, Burton J, Northridge DB, Boon NA, Newby DE; Scottish Aortic Stenosis and Lipid Lowering Therapy, Impact on Regression trial Investigators. Progressive coronary calcification despite intensive lipid-lowering treatment: a randomised controlled trial. *Heart* 2006; 92: 1207-12.

[101] Terry JG, Carr JJ, Kouba EO, Davis DH, Menon L, Bender K, Chandler ET, Morgan T, Crouse JR 3rd. Effect of simvastatin (80 mg) on coronary and abdominal aortic arterial calcium (from the coronary artery calcification treatment with zocor [CATZ] study). *Am J Cardiol* 2007; 99: 1714-7.

[102] Arad Y, Spadaro LA, Roth M, Newstein D, Guerci AD. Treatment of asymptomatic adults with elevated coronary calcium scores with atorvastatin, vitamin C, and vitamin E: the St. Francis Heart Study randomized clinical trial. *J Am Coll Cardiol* 2005; 46: 166-72.

[103] Nissen SE, Nicholls SJ, Sipahi I, Libby P, Raichlen JS, Ballantyne CM, Davignon J, Erbel R, Fruchart JC, Tardif JC, Schoenhagen P, Crowe T, Cain V, Wolski K, Goormastic M, Tuzcu EM; ASTEROID Investigators. Effect of very high-intensity statin therapy on regression of coronary atherosclerosis: the ASTEROID trial. *JAMA* 2006; 295: 1556-65.

[104] Einstein AJ, Berman DS, Min JK, Hendel RC, Gerber TC, Carr JJ, Cerqueira MD, Cullom SJ, DeKemp R, Dickert NW, Dorbala S, Fazel R, Garcia EV, Gibbons RJ, Halliburton SS, Hausleiter J, Heller GV, Jerome S, Lesser JR, Raff GL, Tilkemeier P, Williams KA, Shaw LJ. Patient-centered imaging: shared decision making for cardiac imaging procedures with exposure to ionizing radiation. *J Am Coll Cardiol* 2014; 63: 1480-9.

[105] Achenbach S, Marwan M, Ropers D, Schepis T, Pflederer T, Anders K, Kuettner A, Daniel WG, Uder M, Lell MM. Coronary computed tomography angiography with a consistent dose below 1 mSv using prospectively electrocardiogram-triggered high-pitch spiral acquisition. *Eur Heart J* 2010; 31: 340-6.

[106] Buechel RR, Husmann L, Herzog BA, Pazhenkottil AP, Nkoulou R, Ghadri JR, Treyer V, von Schulthess P, Kaufmann PA. Low-dose computed tomography coronary angiography with prospective electrocardiogram triggering: feasibility in a large population. *J Am Coll Cardiol* 2011; 57: 332-6.

[107] Fuchs TA, Stehli J, Bull S, Dougoud S, Clerc OF, Herzog BA, Buechel RR, Gaemperli O, Kaufmann PA. Coronary computed tomography angiography with model-based iterative reconstruction using a radiation exposure similar to chest X-ray examination. *Eur Heart J* 2014; 35: 1131-6.

[108] Stehli J, Fuchs TA, Bull S, Clerc OF, Possner M, Buechel RR, Gaemperli O, Kaufmann PA. Accuracy of coronary CT angiography using a submillisievert fraction of radiation exposure: comparison with invasive coronary angiography. *J Am Coll Cardiol* 2014; 64: 772-80.

[109] Solomon R. Contrast-induced nephropathy: update with special emphasis on patients with diabetes. *Curr Diab Rep*. 2007 Dec;7(6):454-8.

[110] Mehran R, Aymong ED, Nikolsky E, Lasic Z, Iakovou I, Fahy M, Mintz GS, Lansky AJ, Moses JW, Stone GW, Leon MB, Dangas G. A simple risk score for prediction of contrast-induced nephropathy after percutaneous coronary intervention: development and initial validation. *J Am Coll Cardiol* 2004; 44: 1393-9.

[111] Trivedi HS, Moore H, Nasr S, Aggarwal K, Agrawal A, Goel P, Hewett J. A randomized prospective trial to assess the role of saline hydration on the development of contrast nephrotoxicity. *Nephron Clin Pract* 2003; 93: C29-34.

[112] Komatsu S, Kamata T, Imai A, Ohara T, Takewa M, Miyaji K, Yoshida J, Kodama K. Controlling intracoronary CT number for coronary CT angiography. *J Cardiol* 2013; 61: 155-61.

[113] Kawaguchi N, Kurata A, Kido T, Nishiyama Y, Kido T, Miyagawa M, Ogimoto A, Mochizuki T. Optimization of coronary attenuation in coronary computed tomography angiography using diluted contrast material. *Circ J* 2014; 78: 662-70.

[114] Greenland P, Alpert JS, Beller GA, Benjamin EJ, Budoff MJ, Fayad ZA, Foster E, Hlatky MA, Hodgson JM, Kushner FG, Lauer MS, Shaw LJ, Smith SC Jr, Taylor AJ, Weintraub WS, Wenger NK, Jacobs AK; American College of Cardiology Foundation/American Heart Association Task Force on Practice Guidelines. 2010 ACCF/AHA guideline for assessment of cardiovascular risk in asymptomatic adults: a report of the American College of Cardiology Foundation/American Heart Association Task Force on Practice Guidelines. *Circulation* 2010; 122: e584-636.

[115] American College of Cardiology Foundation Task Force on Expert Consensus Documents, Mark DB, Berman DS, Budoff MJ, Carr JJ,

Gerber TC, Hecht HS, Hlatky MA, Hodgson JM, Lauer MS, Miller JM, Morin RL, Mukherjee D, Poon M, Rubin GD, Schwartz RS. ACCF/ACR/AHA/NASCI/SAIP/SCAI/SCCT 2010 expert consensus document on coronary computed tomographic angiography: a report of the American College of Cardiology Foundation Task Force on Expert Consensus Documents. *Circulation* 2010; 121: 2509-43.

Biographical Sketch

Name: Kohichiro Iwasaki

Affiliation: Department of Cardiology, Okayama Kyokuto Hospital.

Education: Okayama University Graduates School of Medicine and Dentistry, Okayama, 1974-1980.

Address: 567-1 Kurata Nakaku, Okayama City 703-8265 Japan.

Research and Professional Experience:

Coronary intervention, Coronary pressure measurement, Cardiac computed tomography.

Professional Appointments:

Director, Department of Cardiology, Cardiovascular Center, Sakakibara Hospital, Okayama, Okayama, Japan, 1992-2005b.

Clinical Associate Professor, Okayama University Graduates School of Medicine and Dentistry, Okayama, 2000-2005b.

Chairman, Department of Cardiovascular Medicine, Okayama Central Hospital, Okayama, Okayama, Japan, 2005-2010b.

Director, Department of Cardiology, Okayama Kyokuto Hospital, Okayama, Okayama, Japan, 2010-b.

Honors:

Marquis Who's Who in the World 2009.

Marquis Who's Who in Medicine and Healthcare 2009-2010.

Marquis Who's Who in the World 2010.

Marquis Who's Who in the World 2011.

Marquis Who's Who in Science and Engineering 2011-2012.

Marquis Who's Who in the World 2012.

Marquis Who's Who in the World 2013.

Marquis Who's Who in the World 2014.

Publications Last 3 Years:

1. Iwasaki K, Kusachi S. Multidetector computed tomography as a potential modality to detect subclinical atherosclerosis. Coronary Artery Disease, Cardiac Arrest and Bypass Surgery Nova Science Publishers, Inc. New York, 2012: 49-82.
2. Iwasaki K. Myocardial ischemia is a key factor in the management of stable coronary artery disease. World J Cardiol 2014; 6: 130-139.
3. Iwasaki K, Matsumoto T. Characteristics of subclinical coronary artery disease in diabetic patients without known coronary artery disease. Journal of Research in Diabetes Vol. 2014 (2014), Article ID 322292, DOI: 10.5171/2014.322292.
4. Iwasaki K, Matsumoto T. Coronary artery disease and carotid artery disease progress despite normal lipid levels by standard statin therapy in asymptomatic patients without known coronary artery disease: Implications for statin therapy. Enliven: Clinical Cardiology and Research 2014; 1;1-5.
5. Johnson NP, Tóth GG, Lai D, Zhu H, Açar G, Agostoni P, Appelman Y, Arslan F, Barbato E, Chen SL, Di Serafino L, Domínguez-Franco AJ, Dupouy P, Esen AM, Esen OB, Hamilos M, Iwasaki K, Jensen LO, Jiménez-Navarro MF, Katritsis DG, Kocaman SA, Koo BK, López-Palop R, Lorin JD, Miller LH, Muller O, Nam CW, Oud N, Puymirat E, Rieber J, Rioufol G, Rodés-Cabau J, Sedlis SP, Takeishi Y, Tonino PA, Van Belle E, Verna E, Werner GS, Fearon WF, Pijls NH, De Bruyne B, Gould KL. Prognostic value of fractional flow reserve. Linking physiological severity to clinical outcomes. J Am Coll Cardiol 2014; 64: 1641-1654.
6. Iwasaki K, Haraoka K, Hamaguchi T, Imamura T, Kawada S, Ohno M, Kashihara K. Prevalence of subclinical coronary artery disease in ischemic stroke patients. J Cardiol 2015; 65: 71-5.
7. Kawada S, Hamaguchi T, Kitayama M, Imamura T, Ohno M, Kashihara K, Iwasaki K. Multidetector computed tomography angiography to detect the cause of multiple brain infarctions. J Stroke and Cerebrovasc Dis 2015; 24: 348-353.
8. Iwasaki K. Fractional flow reserve is an essential measure for the management of patients with stable coronary artery disease. pp. 75-96. Horizons in World Cardiovascular Research. Volume 8. Nova Science Publishers, Inc. New York 2015

9. Iwasaki K, Matsumoto T, Hasegawa K. Predictors of high-risk coronary artery disease detected by coronary computed tomographic angiography in diabetic patients without known coronary artery disease. Int J Cardiol 2015; 201:324-325. Epub 2015 Aug 10.
10. Iwasaki K, Matsumoto T, Kawada S. Potential utility of multidetector computed tomography to identify both cardiac embolic sources and coronary artery disease in patients with embolic stroke. Cardiology 2016; 133: 205-10.

INDEX

A

B

D

E

F

G

H

N

O

P

T

U

V